QUEST ONE
ACTIVE LIVING:
A GUIDE TO FITNESS, CONDITIONING AND HEALTH

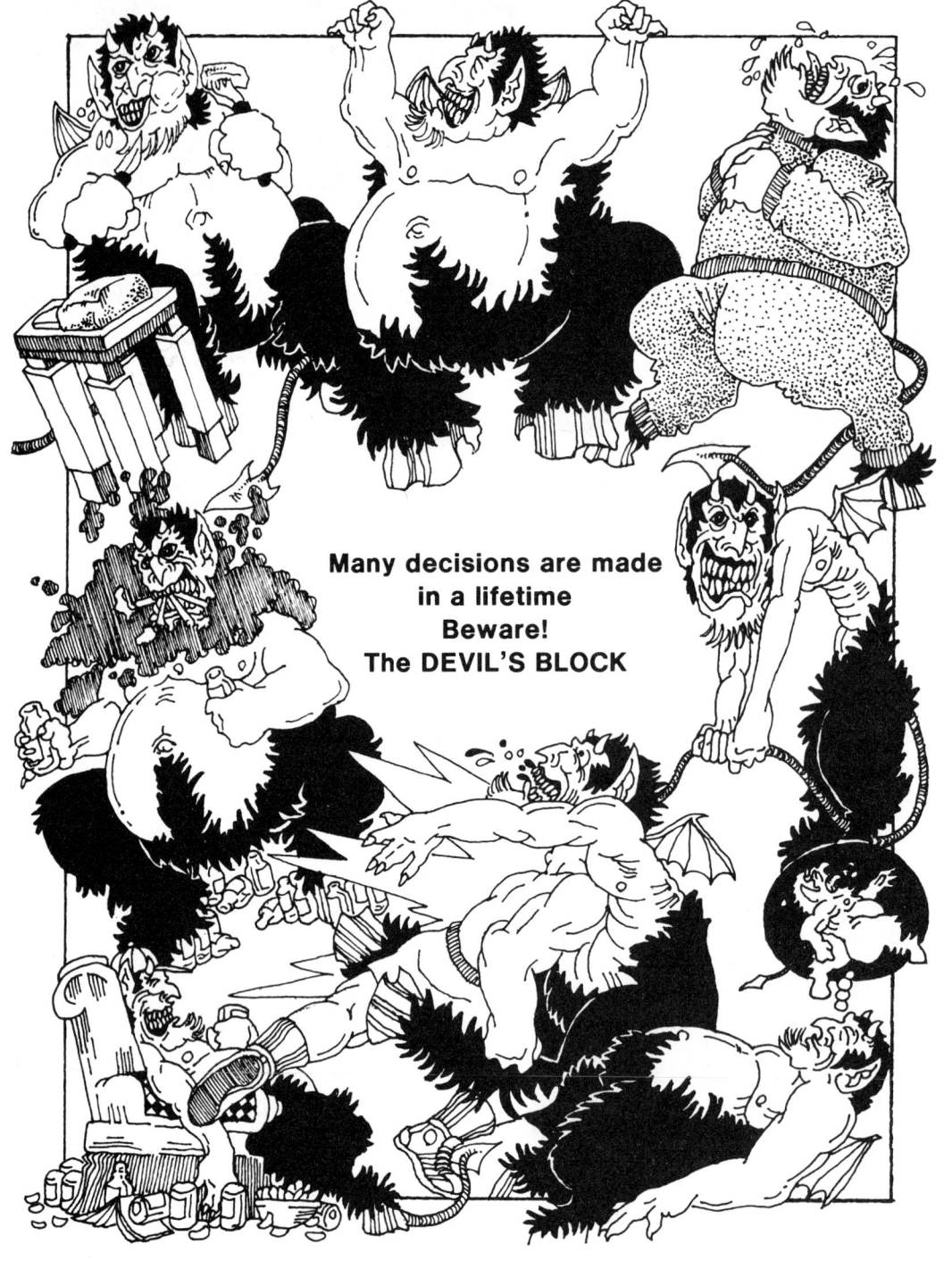

QUEST ONE
ACTIVE LIVING:
A Guide to Fitness, Conditioning and Health

Third Edition

JAMES J. BURD
LEONARD T. SERFUSTINI

Department of Health, Physical Education and Athletics
Glassboro State College

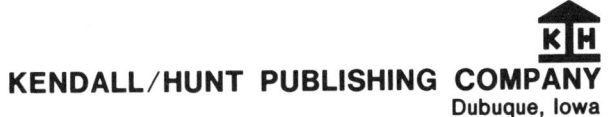

KENDALL/HUNT PUBLISHING COMPANY
Dubuque, Iowa

Copyright © 1976 by James J. Burd and Leonard T. Serfustini

Copyright © 1978, 1981 by Kendall/Hunt Publishing Company

ISBN 0-8403-2520-7

All rights reserved. No part of this publication may be reproduced, stored in a retrieval system, or transmitted, in any form or by any means, electronic, mechanical, photocopying, recording, or otherwise, without the prior written permission of the copyright owner.

Involved

Oh passive partner of the T.V. Age
Take a lesson from an older friend's page.
Consider the one-time carefree sport
Who wishes himself another sort.
He flicks his ashes to the floor
Puffs once, twice, and once more,
Saunters slowly as he's done before,
Reels his beer-bellied body to the door.
"Gymnasium" he cries, "look at me, a loser
Make me strong, a hulk, a bruiser."
The walls echo back the empty plea.

Endure those momentary aches and pains,
Renew your life, review that aim,
Explore the rhythm, lessen the strife,
That daily routine will alter your life.

    William Kushner
    Department of Speech and Theatre
    Glassboro State College

Contents

Foreword, Mark M. Chamberlain ... ix
Acknowledgments ... xi
Forward to New Horizons ... xiii

    1. The Challenge Is Yours ... 1
        Personal Appraisal 1—Attitude Toward Active Living
    2. Active Living and You ... 13
        Personal Appraisal 2—Body Image

Section I: Concepts of Conditioning ... 27

Primary Components of Conditioning ... 28

    3. Cardio-Respiratory Capacity ... 29
        Personal Appraisal 3—Cardio-Respiratory Capacity
    4. Flexibility ... 51
        Personal Appraisal 4—Flexibility
    5. Muscular Strength ... 61
        Personal Appraisal 5—Muscular Strength
    6. Muscular Endurance ... 71
        Personal Appraisal 6—Muscular Endurance

Secondary Components of Conditioning ... 81

    7. Motor Performance Abilities ... 82
        Personal Appraisal 7—Speed
        Personal Appraisal 8—Coordination
        Personal Appraisal 9—Agility
        Personal Appraisal 10—Balance
        Personal Appraisal 11—Explosive Power

Major Influences on Conditioning ... 115

    8. Posture and Body Mechanics ... 116
        Personal Appraisal 12—Posture and Body Mechanics
    9. Nutrition—Weight Control ... 129
        Personal Appraisal 13—Obesity
        Personal Appraisal 14—Body Weight and Caloric Balance
    10. Emotional and Psychological Values ... 161
    11. Chemical Influences and Conditioning ... 165

Profile Chart—Profile of Individual's Results in the Thirteen Self-Appraisal Tests ... 170

Section II: Core Conditioning Program ... 173

    12. Preventive Maintenance ... 175
    13. Flexibility Method of Conditioning ... 182
        Program Experience I
    14. Aerobic/Anaerobic Method of Conditioning ... 190
        Program Experience II
    15. Progressive Resistance Method of Conditioning ... 200
        Program Experience III
        18-Minute Wonder Workout

Section III: Spectrum of Sports Activities ... 223

    16. Introduction to Competition ... 224
    17. Analysis of the Sport Activities ... 229
        Interpretation—Sports Activities Analysis Chart
        Personal Appraisal 15-Individualized Activity Program
    18. The End to What We Hope Will Be the Beginning ... 243

Glossary ... 249

Foreword

During the past twenty years, we in this country have experienced a remarkable awakening of interest in personal physical fitness. Our tennis courts are filled, joggers and bicyclists move through our parks and along our roadways. Swimming pools are crowded. Health clubs and fitness salons abound. In the public schools the role of physical education has been expanded. Hopefully, the sedentary American is again recognizing the great truth that personal well-being requires a sound mind and a healthy body.

But there is no easy route to physical fitness. The dream of a magic pill or a two-minute per week exercise schedule is just that—a dream. The individual who wishes to gain, regain or maintain a high level of personal physical well-being must be prepared to expend both time and effort to attain this goal. This book describes a process by which personal fitness can be attained; it holds out no false promises that the process will be easy.

The goal of physical fitness is well worth the cost. Increasingly we have become aware that the human body must be well-maintained if we are to reduce the probability of cardiovascular disease. Increasingly, we have become aware that good health is not alone the responsibility of the medical profession; rather it is also an individual responsibility which each of us must assume. There is also a growing body of evidence pointing towards the conclusion that physical fitness and mental fitness are closely associated. Human beings are not separable into minds and bodies but rather the mind and the body are so inextricably linked that good or poor health of one immediately affects the other. For our general good health, both physical and mental, a trained and well-conditioned body is requisite.

No book can provide the impetus, the motivation, to make a physical fitness plan work for you. But on the following pages you will find a plan and a process that will enable you to attain your goals of physical and mental fitness. The authors have done their work well—the rest is up to you. I can assure you from direct and personal experience: the plan works, the goals can be attained and the gain is well worth the cost. Don't take my word for it; try it yourself—today.

Mark M. Chamberlain, President
Glassboro State College

Acknowledgments

We would like to express our gratitude to the following, who became "Team Members" and chose to devote a great deal of their time and effort toward our common goal:

To our wives, Barbara and Clyde, whose patience, understanding and encouragement came when we needed it most.

Cathy Barratt proved to be an astute listener and contributor during the many changes and revisions and typed them endlessly into recognizable form. Dr. William Kushner, who recently made Active Living a Way of Life and who became our most persistent critical reader. He also provided us with the poem, *Involved,* which strikes at the heart of our beliefs.

We thank our two young models, Vickie Shaughnessy and Bill Emery, for their vivid poses illustrating a number of exercises. The general illustrations were drawn by Charles Pickford. Andy Prendimano brought our Devil's Block to Life through his artistic talents.

It is with great satisfaction that we complete this text incorporating forty-five years of combined teaching and a lifetime of participation in sports. But, perhaps, most importantly, we realized the true meaning of our text through those who became part of our cohesive team. That philosophy is, we can assist one another in making the "active life" a way of life for all of us. It is the essence of our "first quest."

FORWARD TO NEW HORIZONS

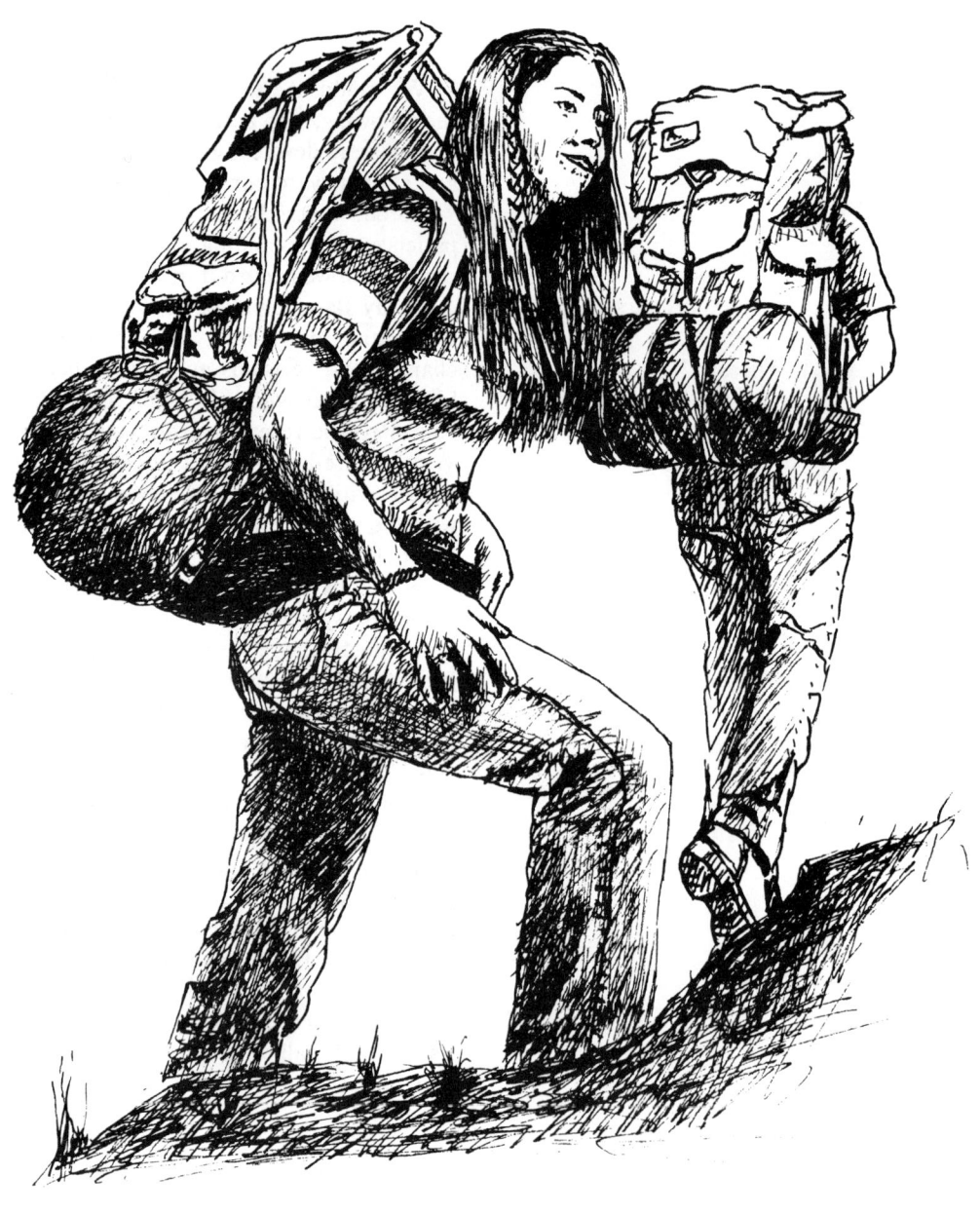

Forward to New Horizons

Our primary objective is to come in contact with all students and, under skillful guidance, assist them in developing an appreciation of Health and Physical Education as a "Way of Life." We hope our readers will adopt a positive attitude toward the value of participation in physical activity so that they will seek further information, participation, and control over their personal state of fitness and health.

We will stress the acquisition of knowledge and concepts in Healthful-Active Living. As students gain knowledge, they will begin to understand their personal state of emotional and physical fitness through experimenting in personal appraisals.

The students will also be exposed to and actively involved in a core program of activity designed to improve the cardiovascular, articulation, and muscular systems. This core activity program is the basis for building high levels of conditioning. Upon completion of this program, having realized increased conditioning levels and understanding basic facts and concepts, the students will become involved in a number of activities selected from the broad spectrum of sport offerings. Students will be encouraged to accept the challenge of new activities, and strive to reach high levels of skill development. We believe the combination of core and sport activities will provide personal satisfaction and enjoyable means of contributing to the development of high levels of mental and physical conditioning.

Keeping yourself fit is a significant key to success regardless of what your career interest may be. Most importantly, participation must be *fun* if lifelong interest is to be maintained.

It must be understood that there is no residual effect of training on the body over a long period of time. If adequate levels of fitness are to be maintained, physical activity must be undertaken with regularity throughout life.

It is hoped that after completion of this approach to a total active health program, students will seek activity as an enjoyable and healthful "Way of Life"—"For the Remainder of Their Lives."

ACTIVE LIVING
NATURE'S WAY OF LIFE

Our intent and commitment is to motivate you to become physically active. Most importantly, we want you to develop an attitude that values participation in meaningful physical activity—until the active life becomes A-Way-of-Life for you.

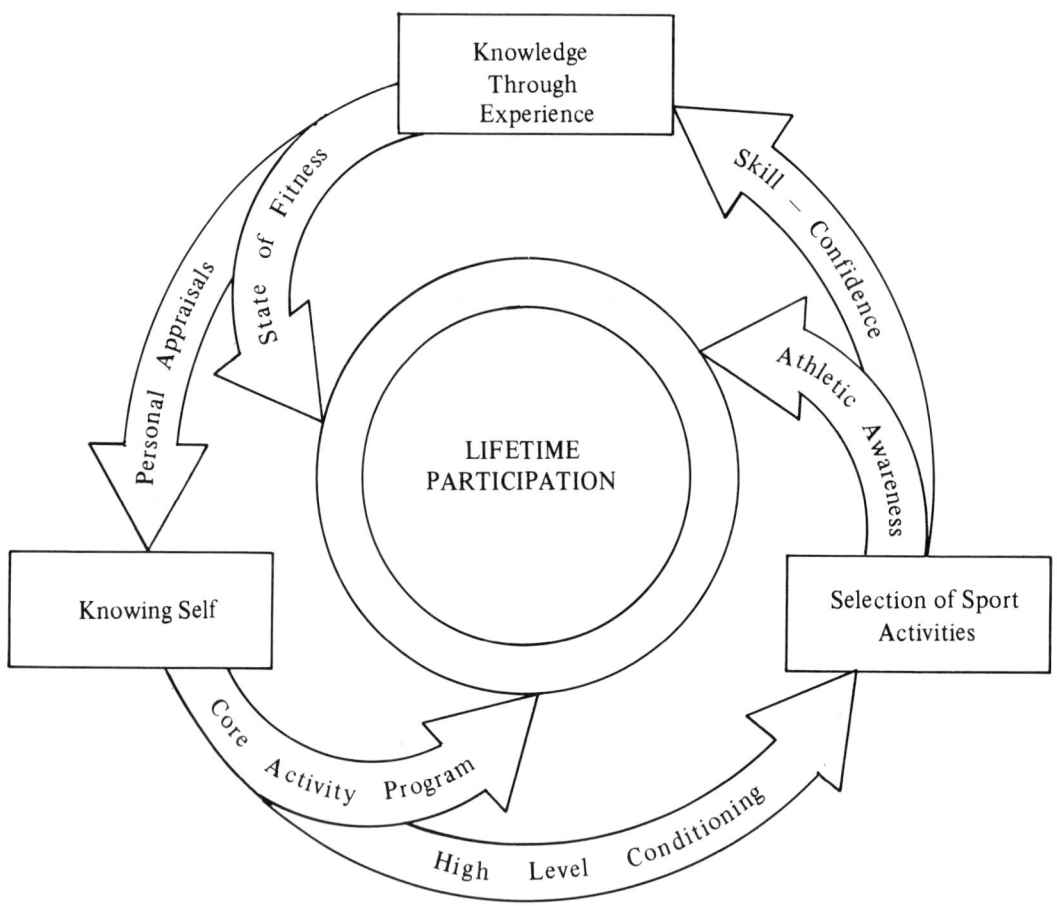

Cycle for—Lifetime Participation

We believe each of us should first become knowledgeable in the concepts of healthful-active living. Experience will be gained through participation in a series of personal appraisals. A means of better knowing self. We hope this insight will inspire action and lead one to become involved in personally satisfying activity. When this occurs, the bridge will have been traversed in developing positive attitudes towards participation and individuals will seek a lifetime of activity.

1
THE CHALLENGE IS YOURS

Science, as well as experience, has provided us with countless reasons for remaining physically active. Therefore, we want to present you with a personal challenge:

You know how you feel./You know how you react to vigorous activity./Your doctor knows the state of your health./Everyone knows how you look./What do you intend to do about it? Today? Tomorrow? In the future?

Critical Assumption

Physical activity is a basic need of the human body. When movement is restricted, the degenerative process begins: muscles atrophy; range of motion or flexibility decreases; and the systems of the body become ineffective. Vigorous physical activity, as a basic human need, is vital to the improvement and maintenance of efficient and healthy bodies.

Are you satisfied with your present state of physical fitness? Does your lifestyle include vigorous physical activity? We invite you to join us and discover the *"why and how"* of planning and participating in programs which are best suited for "you." Programs which will improve and maintain "human conditioning" during your entire life.

Throughout history, man has used physical activity in a variety of ways which have affected his physical and mental well-being. Primitive man relied almost solely upon muscular strength and cardiorespiratory endurance for survival. Conquest and the will to defend oneself against aggression has caused societies to develop programs of exercise and conditioning in preparation for battle. Man has sought to perfect his physical development and attain high levels of skill in order to compete in sport and athletic contests. These competitive events have created entertainment appeal for large numbers of spectators.

Age of Automation

Through the ages, man has discovered and manufactured countless materials, tools and methods which have resulted in saving time and work. As labor and toil have decreased, so has the general state of man's fitness. This phenomenon is especially evident in the American culture as witnessed during the first half of the twentieth century. We have become an almost totally automated society. Our physical needs are usually satisfied only when we choose to break away from this sedentary life-style and seek vigorous activity. It is unfortunate that participation in physical activity on a regular basis is not valued by most members of our society.

Research has presented massive amounts of evidence that demonstrate the critical need for vigorous activity necessary for optimal physical and mental development of children. Few educators would deny the importance of play in the socialization process of children. When parents understand the need for vigorous play activity, their influence is strong in encouraging children to become actively involved.

The scientific community has also presented a significant amount of evidence which shows the very real importance of activity in positively influencing adult health. Some have neglected the implications of this research. We have convinced ourselves that while others may need activity to maintain their health, it is unnecessary for us. Our lives may appear comfortable while we neglect our basic need for movement. The degenerative process caused by a lack of activity is insidious in that it takes a long period of time to recognize its danger signals, and therefore it is a simple matter for teenagers and adults to fall into the trap of a sedentary life. When this style of living becomes habitual, it is difficult to extricate oneself and reverse the process. The more deconditioned a person becomes, initiating an activity program requires more time, and becomes increasingly difficult.

The Challenge

The following questions become your challenge:

1. Will you accept the value of participation in vigorous physical activity?
2. Can you develop healthy and active patterns of living?
3. Will you persevere when faced with the temptations which cause a regression to the sedentary way of life?

To meet this challenge, we will attempt to stimulate you toward action and activity. We believe that you should become knowledgeable in the underlying concepts of anatomy and physiology. We must understand how the systems of the body function in trained and untrained individuals. It is of critical importance that you have the ability to analyze your own state of fitness and develop logical activity programs suited to your needs.

The text begins with a description of basic concepts concerning the principles of anatomy and physiology. Other areas, such as nutrition and weight control, are discussed in terms of their effect upon health and fitness. With this knowledge, you will have taken the first step towards establishing realistic goals and entering into a lifetime of pleasurable activity.

We feel that all people have a need, at some point during their lives, to experience the high levels of conditioning such as those achieved by the varsity athlete. Upon completion of a vigorous workout, many people express the feeling of euphoria. Why not get "high on activity"? The very pleasant feeling which accompanies total relaxation can be experienced at the end of exercise. A sense of well-being and self-fulfillment accompanies high levels of conditioning. As you reach this state, you will have improved ability to adapt to stress and tension. To those who have experienced these sensations, total involvement in vigorous activity programs will become attractive. Section II encourages you to engage in programs specifically designed to produce high levels of conditioning resulting in the effects described above.

One of the principles of physical fitness is that conditioning will deteriorate as activity is decreased or terminated. Wouldn't it be wonderful if once maximum conditioning were realized, it would remain with us for the rest of our lives. But unfortunately this is not the case. For most of us, our state of fitness has gradually decreased from the time of childhood. To a great extent, this is due to a reduction in our physical activity. While some, such as the varsity athlete, may have experienced high levels of conditioning, in most cases, these levels of fitness have rapidly decreased upon the termination of their high school or college athletic career.

Few of us have designed lifetime activity programs that will increase or maintain high levels of condition. This is unfortunate since exercise programs may require little time, can be extremely enjoyable, and most importantly, provide a multitude of health-related benefits.

The third section of our text encourages you to pursue physical activities which suit your needs and interests. In addition, we hope you will develop a confidence and curiosity to seek out new sport skills—forms of sport which may stimulate lifetime interest.

You are encouraged to participate in a variety of physical activities to increase and maintain conditioning levels and guarantee lifelong interest in active living. In this section, physical activities are described and analyzed in terms of the effects they produce in the body.

Summary

Maintaining high levels of conditioning is one of the keys to a successful career and family life. Maintaining fitness can and should be "fun," if lifelong interest is to be realized.

As we begin to understand the importance of physical activity, and personally experience the effects of high levels of conditioning, we can establish realistic and worthwhile goals for ourselves. Through participation in a variety of activities, we may select those that provide the most enjoyable means of realizing these goals. All of us can enjoy vigorous play and should seek out modes of sport that will maintain high levels of fitness, both mental and physical throughout our lives. *Activity for all, and all for activity.*

The Key: Lifelong interest in active living.

Example: "Has been" athletes—the prominent college football star may be an All-American athlete during his tenure as an undergraduate, yet after his senior year, his living pattern may become drastically altered. He moves from the football field to the office. With this transition, his level of physical activity decreases while his caloric requirement diminishes. Unfortunately, he continues to eat the same kind and the same amount of food. Unless our former athlete reduces his food intake, excess calories will be stored as fat. In a short time, his once strong and firm muscles lose tonus and become soft and flabby. In a few years, what was once a superbly conditioned athlete, becomes a middle-aged coronary risk. It is not an athlete who died of heart disease (as is often reported)—it is a former athlete, who like many other victims of heart disease, has become the fat and unfit prey of this great killer.

NOTE: You are now about to embark upon the first in a series of fourteen "Personal Appraisals." These laboratory experiences are designed for "self" evaluation. We have attempted to organize these appraisals in a manner requiring minimal amounts of time and equipment. We hope this will be a significant means to better knowing and understanding yourself. *"The Active Life—Must Be a Way of Life."*

Selected References

Edington, D., and Edgerton, V. *The Biology of Physiology Activity.* Boston: Houghton Mifflin, 1976.

Fleishman, E. A. *The Structure and Measurement of Physical Fitness.* Englewood Cliffs, N.J.: Prentice-Hall, 1964.

Haag, H. *Development and Structure of Astheoretical Framework for Sport Science.* Quest 1979, 31, 25–35.

Kroll, W. *Perspectives in Physical Education.* New York: Academic Press, 1971.

Otto, L., and Alwin, D. *Athletics, Aspirations, and Attainments.* Sociology of Education, 1977. 60, 102–113.

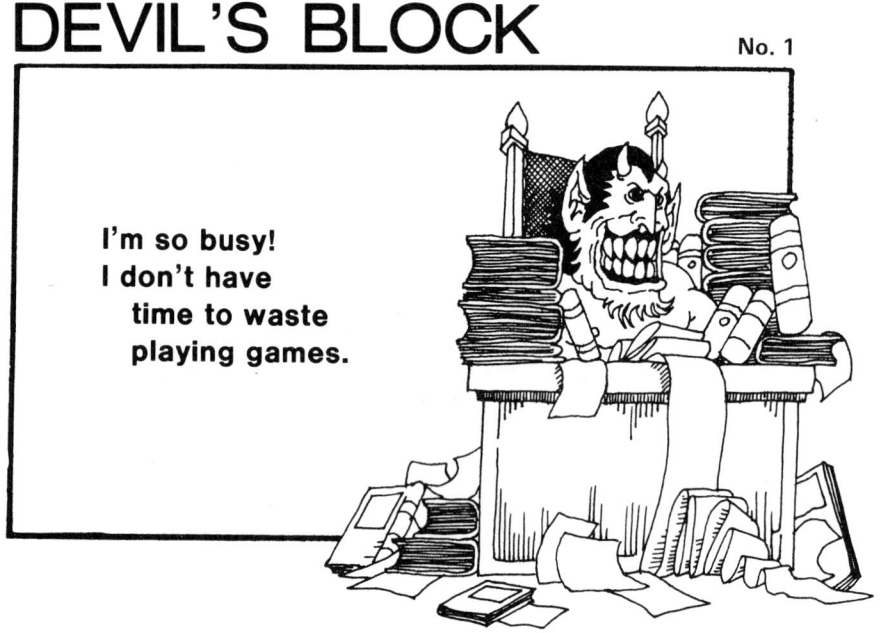

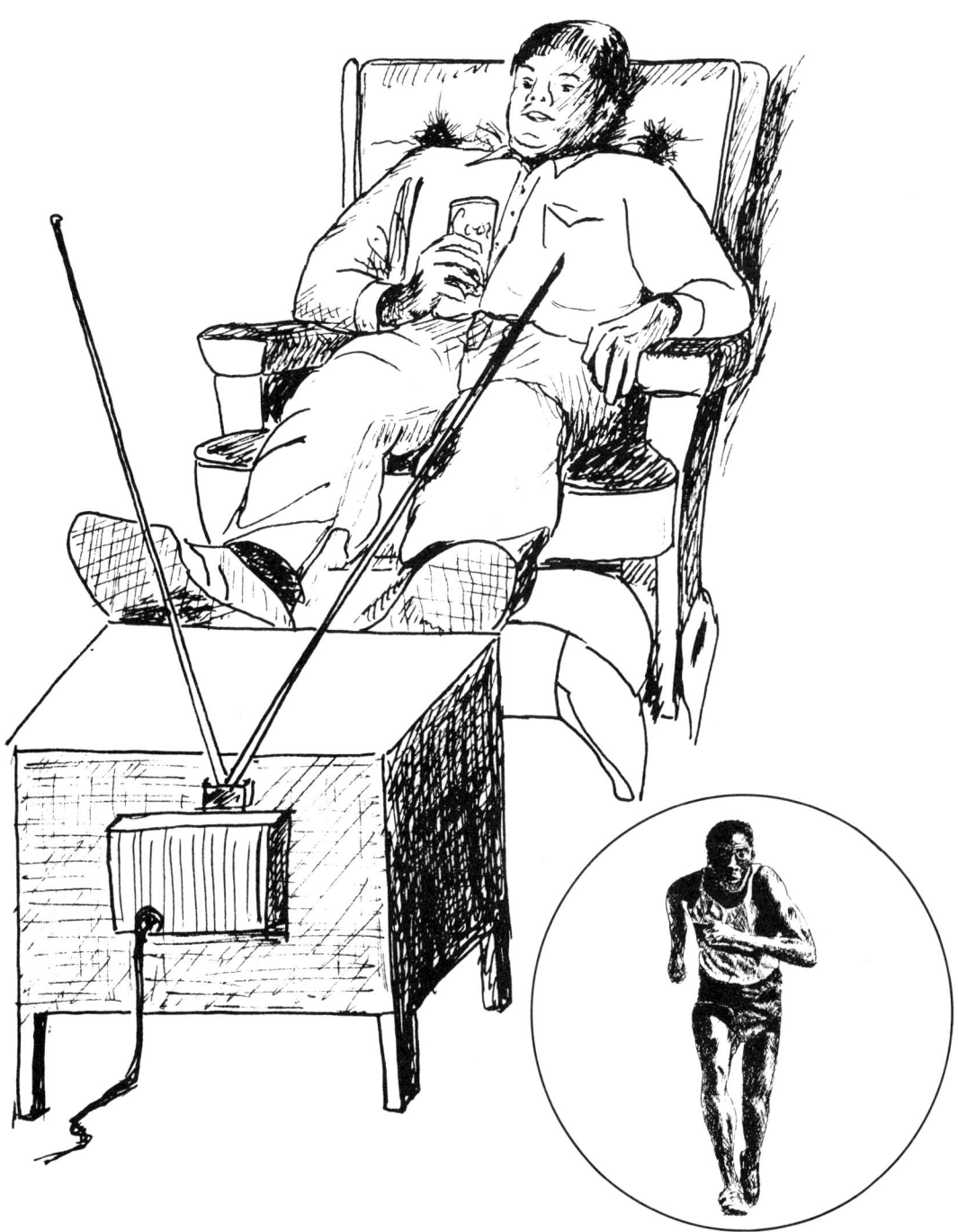

ATTITUDE TOWARD ACTIVE LIVING

PERSONAL APPRAISAL NO. 1
Attitude Toward Active Living

It is important that you make an objective self-analysis of your feelings, attitudes and values that you place upon active living. In attempting this, you can better understand and synthesize your philosophy regarding physical activity. Your attitudes will most likely be reflected in the personal appraisals that follow. We would hope that by the conclusion of this text, those students placing little value on sports and exercise would have altered their philosophies towards seeking out the active life.

Equipment and Facilities

A. Attitude Questionnaire.

Procedures

A. Complete the attitude questionnaire on the following two pages. Note that the number values on the second page are reversed from those on the first page. Do not let this confuse you. If you agree or strongly agree, you will circle a number on the left side of the column. If you disagree or strongly disagree, you will circle a number on the right side of the column. If you have no inclinations in either direction, you will circle the number three.

B. Add the point values on both pages and place the total in the appropriate space at the completion of the questionnaire.

QUESTIONNAIRE

		Strongly Agree				Strongly Disagree
1.	I participate in league competition	5	4	3	2	**(1)**
2.	I enjoy vigorous activity	5	**(4)**	3	2	1
3.	I participate in vigorous activity at least three times per week	5	4	3	2	**(1)**
4.	I feel relaxed after vigorous activity	5	**(4)**	3	2	1
5.	I look forward to vigorous activity	5	**(4)**	3	2	1
6.	I enjoy a variety of types of vigorous activities	5	4	3	**(2)**	1
7.	I feel good when I have been working out	5	**(4)**	3	2	1
8.	Vigorous activity has had a positive effect upon my personal health	5	**(4)**	3	2	1

		Strongly Agree				Strongly Disagree

9. Vigorous activity can contribute to my personal health — (5) 4 3 2 1
10. Vigorous activity is a necessary part of my life style — (5) 4 3 2 1
11. I would recommend vigorous activity for all people — (5) 4 3 2 1
12. Vigorous activity can be enjoyable — (5) 4 3 2 1
13. All people should participate in vigorous activity — (5) 4 3 2 1
14. I looked forward to physical education classes in high school — 5 4 3 (2) 1
15. I appreciated the value of physical education in high school — 5 4 3 (2) 1
16. I successfully participated in physical education in high school — 5 4 3 (2) 1
17. High school physical education contributed to my total health — 5 4 3 (2) 1
18. I participated in interscholastic sports during high school — 5 4 3 (2) 1
19. I enjoy watching sport events on T.V. — 5 (4) 3 2 1
20. I would enjoy participating in league competition — 5 4 3 (2) 1
21. I enjoy attending live sport events — 5 4 3 (2) 1
22. I follow sport events in the news — 5 4 3 (2) 1
23. I enjoy reading sport stories — 5 4 3 (2) 1
24. I associate with people who are involved with vigorous activity — 5 4 3 (2) 1
25. I appreciate other people who participate in vigorous sport activities — 5 (4) 3 2 1
26. I have developed friendships through participation in vigorous activity — 5 4 3 (2) 1
27. I sometimes fantasize that I am a great sport star — 5 (4) 3 2 1
28. People in sports seem to be happy and well-adjusted — 5 (4) 3 2 1
29. I do not look forward to competing in athletic or sport contests — 1 (2) 3 4 5
30. I do not enjoy vigorous activity — 1 2 3 4 (5)
31. I do not enjoy the feeling of fatigue after a workout — 1 (2) 3 4 5
32. I do not participate in league competition — 1 (2) 3 4 5
33. There are very few vigorous activities which I enjoy — 1 (2) 3 4 5
34. I try to avoid exercise whenever I can — 1 2 3 (4) 5
35. Vigorous activity has had a negative effect upon my health — 1 2 3 (4) 5

		Strongly Agree				Strongly Disagree

36. Vigorous activity is unnecessary in my life-style — 1 2 3 (4) 5
37. I cannot recommend vigorous activity to other people — 1 2 3 (4) 5
38. Vigorous activity is not enjoyable — 1 2 3 (4) 5
39. Vigorous activity is unnecessary for most people — 1 2 3 (4) 5
40. I did not look forward to physical education classes in high school — 1 (2) 3 4 5
41. I did not appreciate the value of physical education in high school — 1 (2) 3 4 5
42. I was unsuccessful in physical education during high school — 1 2 3 (4) 5
43. High school physical education did not contribute to my total health — 1 2 3 4 (5)
44. I was not interested in interscholastic sports during high school — (1) 2 3 4 5
45. I do not watch sport contests on T.V. — 1 (2) 3 4 5
46. I would not enjoy participating in league competition — (1) 2 3 4 5
47. I do not attend live sport events — (1) 2 3 4 5
48. I am not interested in following sporting events in the news — (1) 2 3 4 5
49. I do not enjoy reading sport literature — (1) 2 3 4 5
50. I do not associate with people involved with physical activity — (1) 2 3 4 5
51. I do not appreciate people who successfully compete in sport contests — 1 2 3 4 (5)
52. My friends do not participate in vigorous physical activity — 1 (2) 3 4 5
53. I have never desired to be a great sport star — 1 2 3 (4) 5
54. Most people involved with sports do not seem well-adjusted — 1 2 3 (4) 5

Total Score 160

PERSONAL HISTORY OF ACTIVE PARTICIPATION

A. List each of the sports you competed in along with participation in other physical activities which contributed to your fitness during elementary school.

1.
2.
3.
4.
5.
6.
7.
8.

B. List each of the sports you competed in along with participation in other physical activities which contributed to your fitness during junior high school.

1.
2.
3.
4.
5.
6.
7.
8.

C. List each of the sports you competed in along with participation in other physical activities which contributed to your fitness during senior high school.

1.
2.
3.
4.

5.
6.
7.
8.

D. List any additional physical activities that you have engaged in since senior high school.
1.
2.
3.
4.
5.
6.
7.
8.

EVALUATION REPORT
Personal Appraisal No. 1

appreciation evaluation.

Name _____

Date _____

Lifetime Participation

I. *Laboratory Title:* Attitude Toward Active Living

II. *Objective:*

III. *Results:* Total Score _____

The scores will range from 54 to 270. The middle score is 162. Scores falling within the following ranges indicate general descriptions of the values one places on activity.

   54–81 = Gross aversion towards physical activity

  81–108 = Distaste of physical activity

108–134 = Somewhat negative attitude towards physical activity

134–189 = Average values towards physical activity

189–216 = Can see values in physical activity

216–243 = Positive attitude towards activity

243–270 = Places great value on physical activity

IV. *Analysis:*

   1. To what extent do you feel your present life style includes vigorous physical activity? Explain!

   2. In your opinion are the results of this personal appraisal significant? Explain.

3. What experiences have you had which influenced the development of your attitude toward active living?

4. Has the amount of vigorous activity in your life style increased or decreased since high school. Explain why changes have occurred.

V. *Implications*

1. What type of motivation would you need to improve your attitude and participation in vigorous physical activity as a way of life?

2. In future years, what do you envision as your outlet in physical activity.

2
ACTIVE LIVING AND YOU

Ecological Movement

Ecology has become a national priority of our government and the general public. It is with pride and satisfaction that we embrace the tenets of an ecological movement for we see ourselves contributing to the improvement of the environment, and as a direct result a better life for us and for generations to come.

We have at our disposal a vast energy store which can be turned on at any time and yet is relatively inexpensive. This source of energy is the human body with its overwhelming potential for generating energy. In the name of convenience we drive to the mailbox and corner store rather than walk and choose to purchase a menagerie of mechanical and electrical devices which will perform simple physical tasks. An expensive energy source is necessary to operate these devices, yet our body offers us free energy to complete these same tasks with a bonus of improved physiological condition.

A critical concern of the ecological movement is the preservation of our natural resources; there is an aggressive and active ecological movement in our country concerning the pollution of our environment and the senseless waste of our natural resources. Perhaps the greatest ecological problem of all is the unnecessary pollution of our bodies through the intake of chemical substances and the body's deterioration through disuse. In the diseased, injured or deficient states, prescribed drugs can be beneficial—otherwise, they are pollutants.

The body is an incomparable composite of ecological systems which operates its own industrial plants and waste removal facilities. The efficiency of these systems is enhanced through physical activity. Therefore, it is imperative to develop a pride in one's body and respect for the proper functioning of the body's physiological systems.

Our greatest natural resource is the unlimited human potential for solving the great problems of our time and building a world of friendship, love and compassion. The waste of this potential through premature death, illness and disinterest is inexcusable. We have the ability to prevent premature death, eradicate many types of illness, and turn disinterest into productivity. Vigorous lifestyles prolong productive life and enhance a zest for living. We look to the spoilers of earth, yet one of our most unfortunate wastes can be found in the vast numbers of people who allow themselves to degenerate both mentally and physically as they refuse to strive toward their true capacity. What better place to begin conservation than our own bodies, our most precious natural resource.

Pride and satisfaction will result when immersing oneself in the ecology of the human body. This self-improvement and increased efficiency of our personal resources benefit not only ourselves and our families, but our total culture. In this effort, we can become happy, satisfied, and contributing members of society.

The Super-Sapien

Active living is a friend of those who practice it. It is a philosophy, a way of life. When we live actively, we realize a great deal of life's potential. In choosing this style of living, we receive a great deal from life; excitement, satisfaction and health.

Let us present a composite picture of people involved in active living. These individuals recognize their limitations, as well as their strengths, and are willing to seek success within realistic parameters. In accepting themselves, they willingly look for ways to improve while striving towards their full potential. They are knowledgeable regarding health matters and seek information which may assist them in active living. They create and persevere in following activity programs in which they are able to attain personal satisfaction as well as health-related benefits. They are energetic and seem to have a zest for living.

The concept of active living implies that people include vigorous activity in their life-styles which will promote and maintain the quality of their health. These values may be psychological as well as physical. In striving toward this style of living, each of us should attempt to become closely aware of ourselves. We should recognize limitations that heredity, illness, age, etc., may have imposed on us. Most importantly, we should realize the great potential that lies within these parameters, establish realistic goals for ourselves, and begin to live actively as we reach for the attainment of our optimal potential.

Therefore, this text is specifically designed so that each individual student will be able to make an accurate assessment of the following:

1. Personal attitudes toward active living
2. Implications of life-style changes
3. Present state of physical fitness
4. Limitations and potential
5. Establishing worthwhile goals
6. Selection of activity programs
7. Methods of maintaining lifetime fitness

It is of vital importance that each of us lead a physically active life. Not everyone can become a Mr. America or a Ms. America. The All-American and the professional athlete may be unrealistic goals for the vast majority of us. The level of skill and the type of activities are choices that are left up to each individual. The underlying implications are to build and maintain a healthy well-conditioned body.

We are attempting to develop *"Super-Sapiens,"* individuals who reach out to live a full and rewarding life. The "Super-Sapiens" need not become heroes, win accolades, or be voted all-stars. They may not find it necessary to compete with others. They are people who realize the importance of maintaining a positive state of physical and mental health. They structure their lives in a

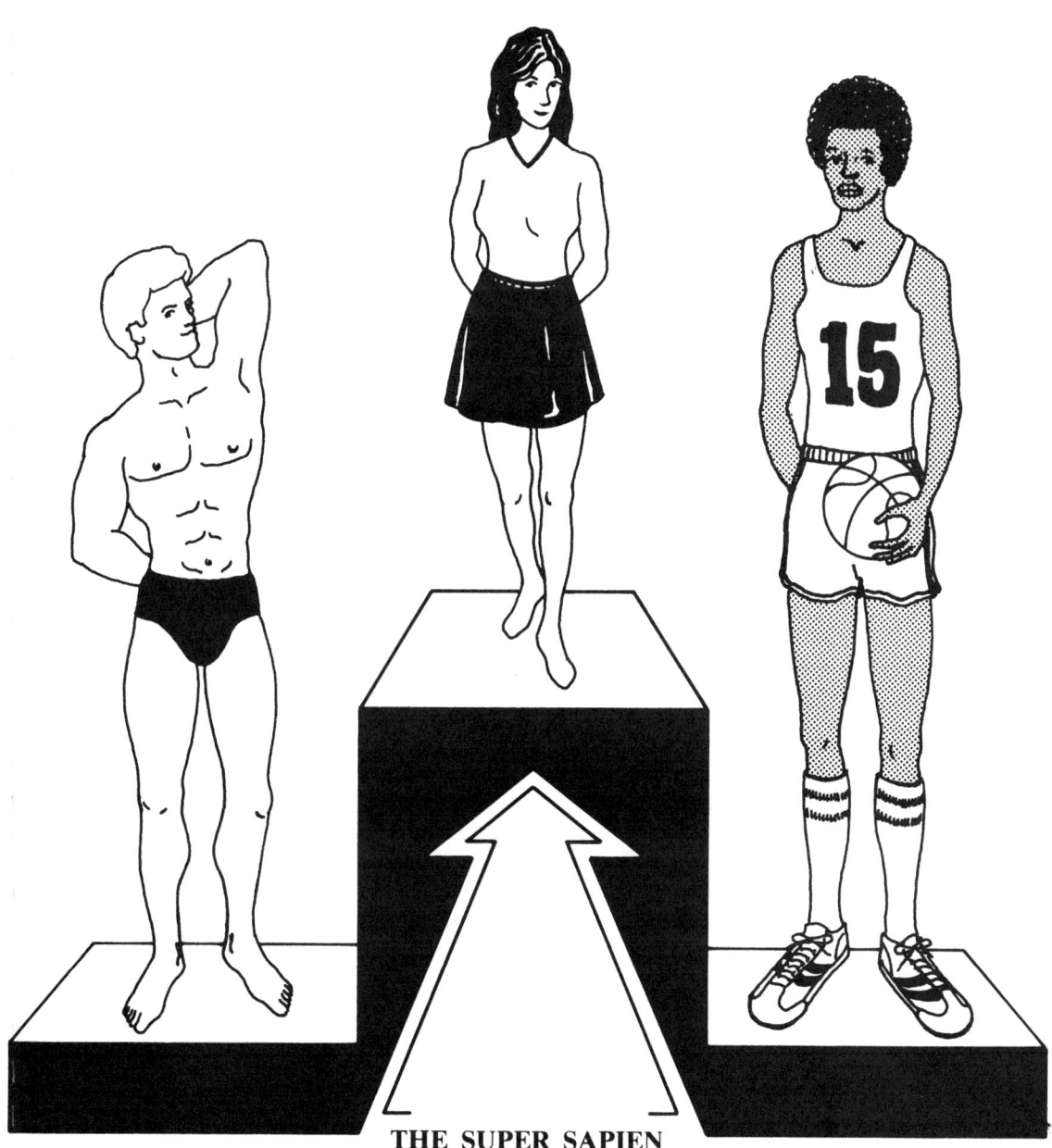

manner which allows them the freedom to be vigorous and active. They are able to cope with the stress and strain of daily living without experiencing undue emotional and physical fatigue. These individuals enjoy life and have a very profound effect upon those around them. They can truly be termed "Super-Sapiens."

Recipe for the Super-Sapien

1. *Able to maintain a resting heart rate below 72 beats per minute*
2. *Able to walk up a flight of stairs without experiencing physical discomfort*
3. *Able to perform light physical activity without noticeably increasing heart rate*
4. *Able to pass a physical examination with flying colors*
5. *Able to meet daily responsibilities without undue fatigue*
6. *Able to look forward to some type of physical activity after the completion of a day's work*
7. *Able to look forward to returning to work after an enjoyable weekend*
8. *Able to resist a second helping at dinnertime*
9. *Able to look into a mirror and appreciate appearance*
10. *Able to make acceptable emotional adjustments to daily problems*
11. *Able to handle stress without producing anxiety*
12. *Able to say no to temptations that have negative values*
13. *Able to make lasting friendships*
14. *Able to accept strengths as well as limitations and strive to become a better person*

From these general facts, concepts have been developed to assist your venture into becoming a Super-Sapien and to also assist you in maintaining this condition.

You are about to embark on a challenging venture; that of becoming a "Super-Sapien" and learning how to maintain this condition throughout life.

Reach out for *your* true potential. Your next step in getting to know yourself is through Personal Appraisal II, "Body Image."

Selected References

Behnke, A. R., and Wilmore, J. H. *Evaluation and Regulation of Body Build and Composition.* Englewood Cliffs, N.J.: Prentice-Hall, 1974.

Jette, M., and Cureton, T. K. Anthropometric and selected motor fitness measurements of men engaged in a long-term program of physical activity. *Research Quarterly,* 1976, 47, 666–671.

Kane, J. E. Personality and Physical Abilities. in G. S. Kenyon (Ed.) *Contemporary Psychology of Sport.* Chicago: Athletic Institute, 1970.

Parizkova, J. Impact of age diet and exercise on man's body composition. *Anals of the New York Academy of Science,* 1963, 110, 661–674.

DEVIL'S BLOCK No. 2

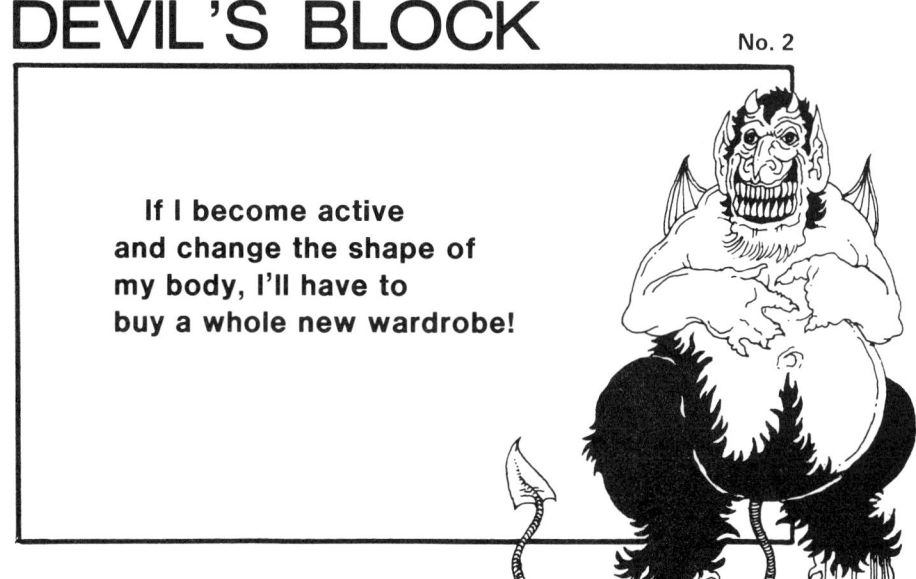

If I become active and change the shape of my body, I'll have to buy a whole new wardrobe!

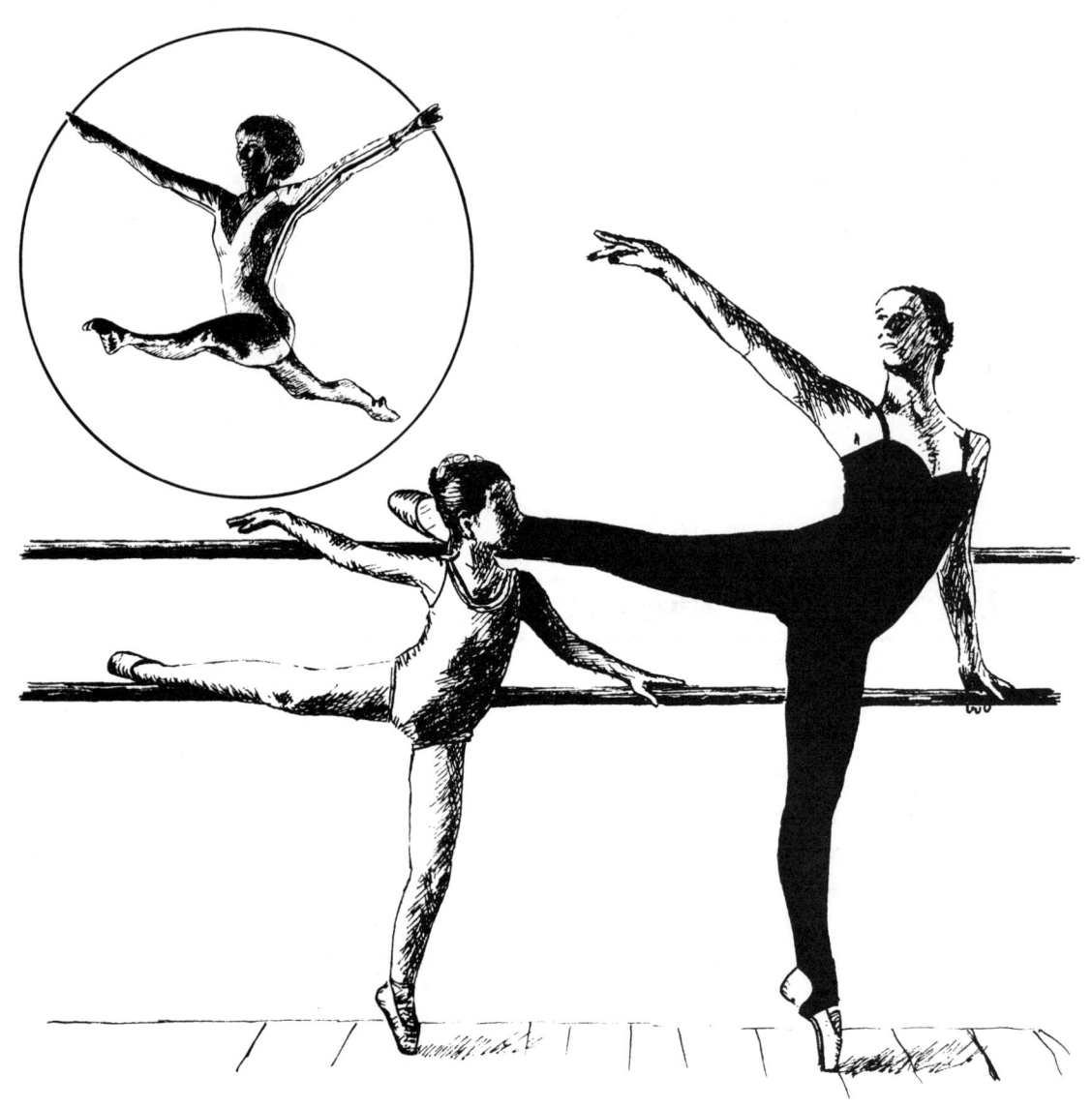

BODY IMAGE

PERSONAL APPRAISAL NO. 2
Body Image

One of the outcomes which may be derived from participation in vigorous physical activity is improved body symmetry. There is no reason why we should not have an honest pride in our bodies. "Body Image" is an integral part of "Self-image," which assists us in the formation of our "Self-concept." This becomes a critical factor in personality development.

An important fringe benefit of exercise is better appearance. Maintaining excellent muscular tonus and reduction of adipose tissue does a great deal to enhance the overall appearance of the body. It is ludicrous to deny we have no interest in this, as our society literally spends millions of dollars annually for assistance in improving appearance. We should have concern for our personal appearance. The quickest, most sustaining and cheapest method of improving appearance is through vigorous physical activity.

We can influence body shape and form through the intelligent use of exercise and proper nutrition since body shape can be altered by:

1. Increasing the size of muscular mass
2. Reduction of adipose tissue
3. A concern for proper posture

Through a properly prescribed program of physical activity, improved body symmetry can be easily obtained. Recording our present body measurements (as a pretest) will assist us in recognizing changes as they occur.

Equipment and Facilities
    A. Tape Measure

Procedures

A. Record Body Measurements
  1. Complete this appraisal while working with a partner
  2. Note the illustration as to the specific points measurements are taken
  3. Do not force the tape. Maintain a consistent firmness throughout all measurements
  4. Record all measurements to the nearest eighth of an inch
  5. All measurements should be taken while body is in a relaxed state

BODY MEASUREMENTS   *assignment*

1. Weight   110
2. Height   5.2'
3. Neck   12
4. Shoulders (girth) 18
5. Bicep (Right)   9.6
6. Bicep (Left)   9.5
7. Forearm (Right) 9.5
8. Forearm (Left)   9.5
9. Chest (Normal)   33
10. Chest (Expanded) 34
11. Waist   28
12. Hips   35
13. Buttocks   38
14. Thigh (Right)   21
15. Thigh (Left)   21
16. Calf (Right)   14
17. Calf (Left)   14
18. Wrist (Right)   6.
19. Wrist (Left)   6.1/4
20. Ankle (Right)   8.
21. Ankle (Left)   8.

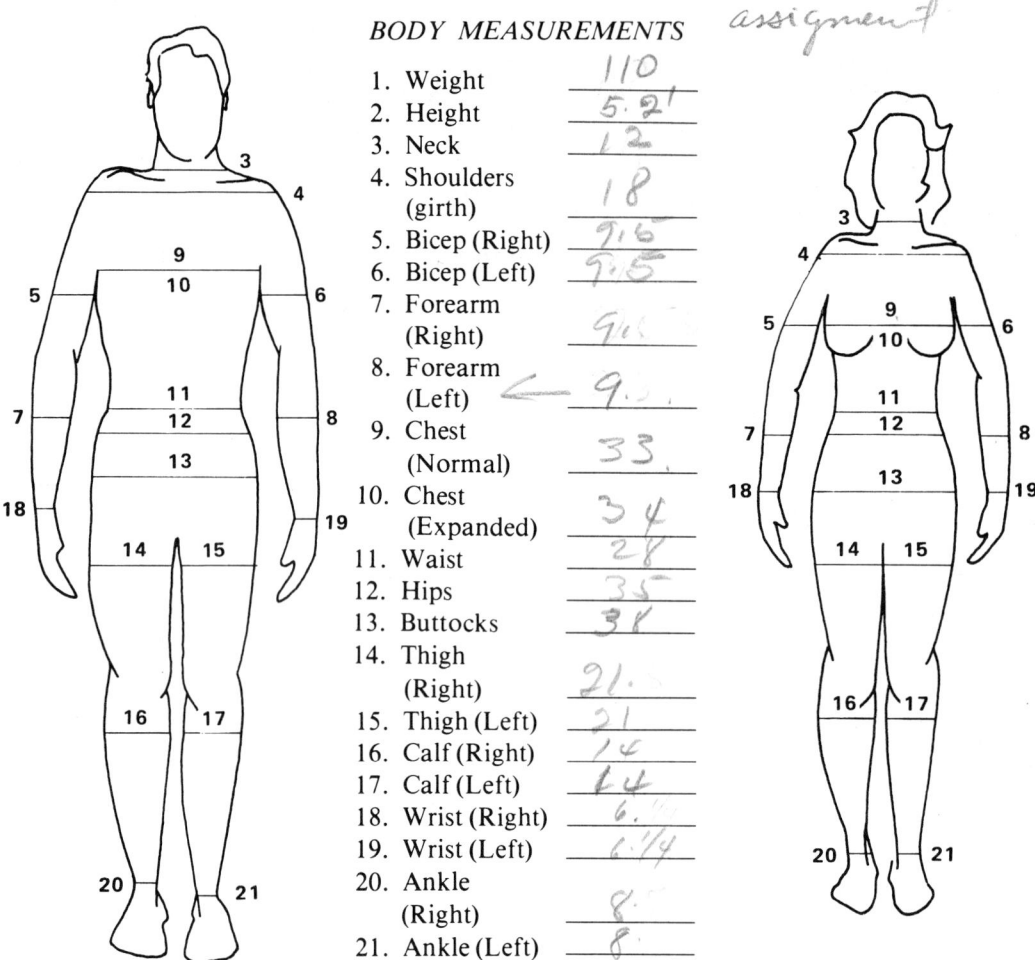

Proportions for Ideal Body Symmetry

A realistic approach to body development is to strive for ideal symmetry. Body symmetry is the key to a more pleasing appearance. The following measurements which show relationships are indicators of ideal body symmetry.

Male

Chest-(normal) Waist (10" min. Difference)
Biceps-Neck-Calf (Same Measurements)
Waist-Thigh-Calf (9" Difference)
Bicep-Forearms (3"–4" Difference)

Female

Bust-Waist (10" Min. Difference)
Bust-Hips (Similar Measurements)
Thigh-Knee-Calf-Ankles (In normal standing position, heels together, toes pointed slightly outward—these four points should touch with space showing in-between)

B. Skeletal Classification

The measurement of the wrist and ankle are usually devoid of muscular mass and adipose tissue. This makes the measurement of these structures an ideal means of determining bone size.

1. The wrist and ankle measurements are quick indicators for size of bone structure
2. Circle the range in which your wrist and ankle measurement falls

Range:	Wrist	Small	Medium	Large
	Female	−5⅛"	5¼"−6⅛"	6¼"+
	Male	−6½"	6⅝"−7⅛"	7¼"+

Range:	Ankle	Small	Medium	Large
	Female	−7½"	7⅝"−8⅞"	9"+
	Male	−8½"	8⅝"−9¾"	9⅞"+

C. Body-type Classification

1. Study the brief description and illustration of body-types
2. Compare your measurements and body shape with others in the class
3. On the basis of this analysis, place a checkmark on the scale indicating your body type

Ectomorph	**Mesomorph**	**Endomorph**
Is thin-muscled and often has light bone structure. The body looks fragile and delicate. Neck and arms are usually long. The shoulders are usually rounded. Weak upper arms and thighs are typical of the extreme ectomorph. There is very little adipose tissue on the body.	Muscular and often heavy bone structure. Noted for excellent muscular tone and development. Possesses a fairly long neck, broad shoulders, large chest, relatively slender waist and broad hips. The arms and legs are well-developed. This person is strong.	Possesses a roundness or a softness to the body. There is little muscle development. The arms and legs show very little muscle development. The weight of this individual is centered in the front of the body around the abdomen. There are heavy pads of fat around the backs of the hips, abdomen, buttocks, thighs and arms.

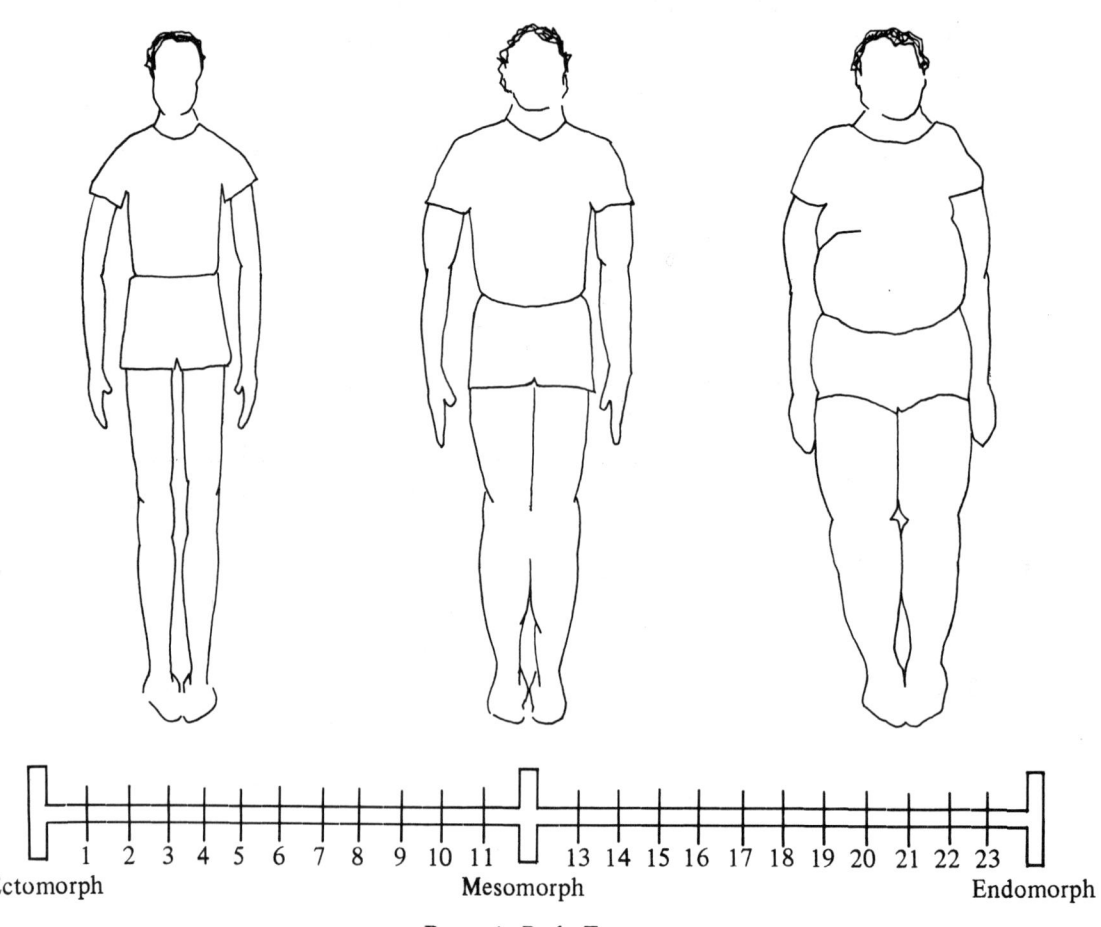

Range in Body-Type

EVALUATION REPORT
Personal Appraisal No. 2

Name _____

Date _____

Lifetime Participation

I. *Laboratory Title:* Body Image

II. *Objective:*

III. *Results:*

    A. Body Measurements:

1. Weight _____	8. Forearm (L) _____	15. Thigh (L) _____
2. Height _____	9. Chest (Nor) _____	16. Calf (R) _____
3. Neck _____	10. Chest (Exp) _____	17. Calf (L) _____
4. Shoulders _____	11. Waist _____	18. Wrist (R) _____
5. Bicep (R) _____	12. Hips _____	19. Wrist (L) _____
6. Bicep (L) _____	13. Buttocks _____	20. Ankle (R) _____
7. Forearm (R) _____	14. Thigh (R) _____	21. Ankle (L) _____

    B. Skeletal Classification: Wrist _____ Ankle _____

    C. Body-type: _____ Number: _____

Rate your body image on the basis of your findings:

Rating	Classification
1	Excellent
2	Above average
3	Average
4	Below average
5	Poor

IV. *Analysis:*

1. Do the results of this personal appraisal substantiate or contradict your feelings of self concept? Explain.

2. List and describe areas of body image, shape and size that you feel are acceptable.

3. In view of the results of A, B and C, how would you rate your body shape, size and image?

4. List and describe areas in which you feel you need improvement.

V. *Implications:*

1. Describe the activities that you are interested in which will enhance or improve your body image.

2. Explain how an improved body may influence your life!

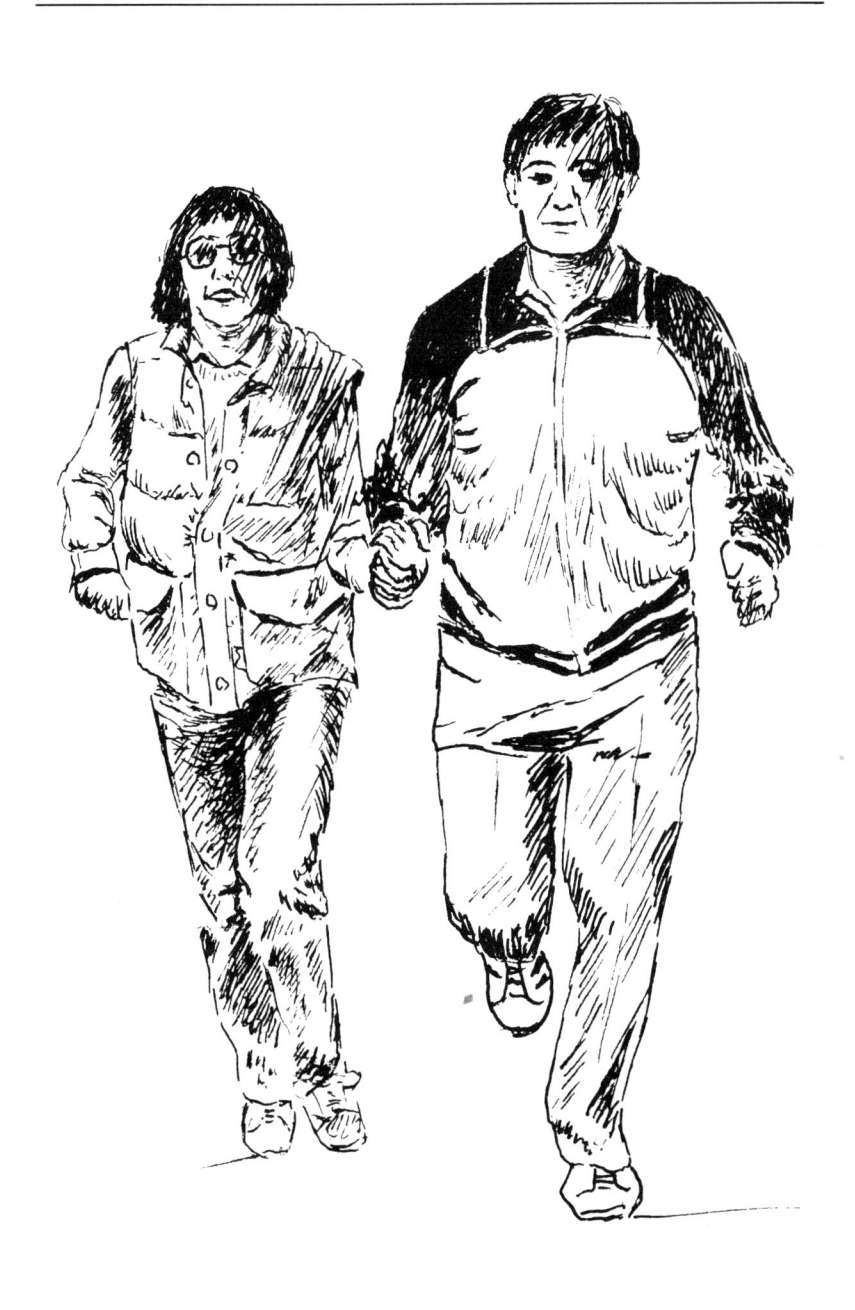

SECTION 1—CONCEPTS OF CONDITIONING

Section I

CONCEPTS OF CONDITIONING

The meaning of total physical fitness should be clear before the essential components of conditioning are identified. Physical fitness can be defined as the ability to carry out daily tasks with vigor and alertness, without undue fatigue, and with ample energy to enjoy leisure-time pursuits and to meet unusual situations and unforeseen emergencies. Thus, physical fitness is the ability to endure, to bear up, to cope with stress, and to persevere under difficult circumstances. This definition implies that physical fitness is more than simply "not being ill" or merely, "being well." It is a positive quality, extending on a continuum from failing health and death to an abundant life of satisfaction and personal wellbeing. Individuals have some degree of physical fitness; it varies considerably in different people and in the same person from time to time. It may be considered minimal in the severely ill and maximal in the highly trained athlete. In as much as this physical fitness objective is so general, a breakdown into its underlying components is essential for its measurement and for determining the appropriate program content to achieve the full realization of total fitness and conditioning.

This section is primarily concerned with the analysis of a number of topics that are affected by and to some extent affect the conditioning process. These areas vary in many respects, but can be grouped into three categories.

The initial segment (Chapters 3, 4, 5 and 6) is called "The Primary Components" of conditioning. This area considers cardio-respiratory capacity, flexibility, muscular strength and muscular endurance. These components are classified as primary since they are the most influential aspects affecting the conditioning process. In addition, they are of major importance in the control of degenerative disease and the maintenance of positive health.

The second segment (Chapter 7) is labeled, "The Secondary Components" of conditioning. This area discusses speed, coordination, agility, balance and explosive power. These qualities, while being of extreme importance to the proficiency of the athlete, will usually receive little attention from the average person.

The final segment, (Chapters 8, 9, 10, 11) "the major influences" upon conditioning, investigates body mechanics, weight control, chemical influences and emotional adjustments. These topics are closely related to the conditioning process and play a critical role in influencing the state of our physical and mental health.

PRIMARY COMPONENTS OF CONDITIONING

Chapter 3　　Cardio-Respiratory Fitness
　　　　　　　Personal Appraisal No. 3
Chapter 4　　Flexibility
　　　　　　　Personal Appraisal No. 4
Chapter 5　　Muscular Strength
　　　　　　　Personal Appraisal No. 5
Chapter 6　　Muscular Endurance
　　　　　　　Personal Appraisal No. 6

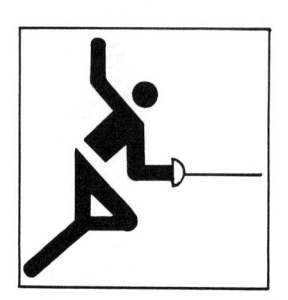

3

CARDIO-RESPIRATORY CAPACITY

The ability of the human organism in meeting life's demands is directly related to the state of functional efficiency of the cardio-respiratory system. Cardio-respiratory capacity refers to the ability of the heart, vascular system and lungs to respond to life's requirements for energy, nutrition and waste removal. Cardio-respiratory capacity is characterized by muscular contractions for relatively long periods of time, during which maximal adjustments of the cardio-respiratory system become necessary. The capacity of the cardio-respiratory system in adjusting to exercise demands, is a key factor in athletic proficiency. This state of functional efficiency is crucial for each of us when it becomes a factor in our ability to resist the onset of degenerative heart disease.

The cardio-respiratory system composed of the blood, heart, vascular bed and lungs functions primarily as a transport system. It conveys necessary materials such as glucose and oxygen to the cells, and the end products of metabolism such as carbon dioxide and lactic acid from the cells.

Circulatory System

The blood, heart and vascular bed are the primary components of the circulatory system.

1. Blood—This liquid is composed of a variety of substances which have varied functions. Nutrients, such as glucose, lipids and amino acids, are destined for the cells. These along with other dissolved solids, such as enzymes, antibodies, hormones, fibrinogen, albumin, globulins and certain waste products circulate throughout the body as components of the bloods' plasma. The cellular portion of the blood is composed of red blood cells, white blood cells and platelets. One of the primary functions of red blood cells is to transport oxygen to body tissue and remove carbon dioxide. The white blood cells fight infection while the platelets are involved in the clotting process.

2. Heart—This muscular organ functions as a pump in which blood is forced throughout the entire body. This provides the cells with nourishment in the form of dissolved foodstuffs and oxygen and also allows for the removal of carbon dioxide and other waste materials. The heart is a muscle with innate rhythmic contractions. It requires a rich blood supply (coronary arteries) in order to meet its metabolic requirements.

3. Vascular Bed—The vascular bed is composed of the arteries, small arteries, arterioles and capillaries which lead to the tissues where the exchange of oxygen, carbon dioxide, nutrients and waste products occur. The arterial walls contain involuntary or smooth muscle which enables them to constrict or dilate. A change in the diameter of these walls produces a dramatic change in the systemic blood pressure and a corresponding adjustment in blood flow to specific parts of the body. The vascular bed also includes the venules and veins which transport deoxygenated blood back to the heart and lungs for oxygenation.

Respiratory System

Respiration occurs on four levels:

1. Ventilation or breathing, in which gases enter and leave the lungs.
2. External respiration in which oxygen passes from the alveoli of the lungs into the capillaries, and carbon dioxide passes from the capillaries of the lung into the alveoli.
3. Internal respiration in which oxygen and carbon dioxide are exchanged between the capillaries and the cells.
4. True respiration which is the oxidative process within the cells.

The lungs are composed of a system of tubes gradually decreasing in diameter. The smallest tubes or bronchioles are surrounded by minute structures called alveoli through which gas exchange takes place. The contraction of the diaphragm and intercostal muscles cause an enlargement of the chest cavity, resulting in a decreased pressure which allows the lungs to expand and inspiration of oxygen to occur. Upon relaxation of these muscle groups, expiration occurs allowing carbon dioxide and other gases to leave the lungs.

MAJOR STRUCTURES OF THE VASCULAR BED

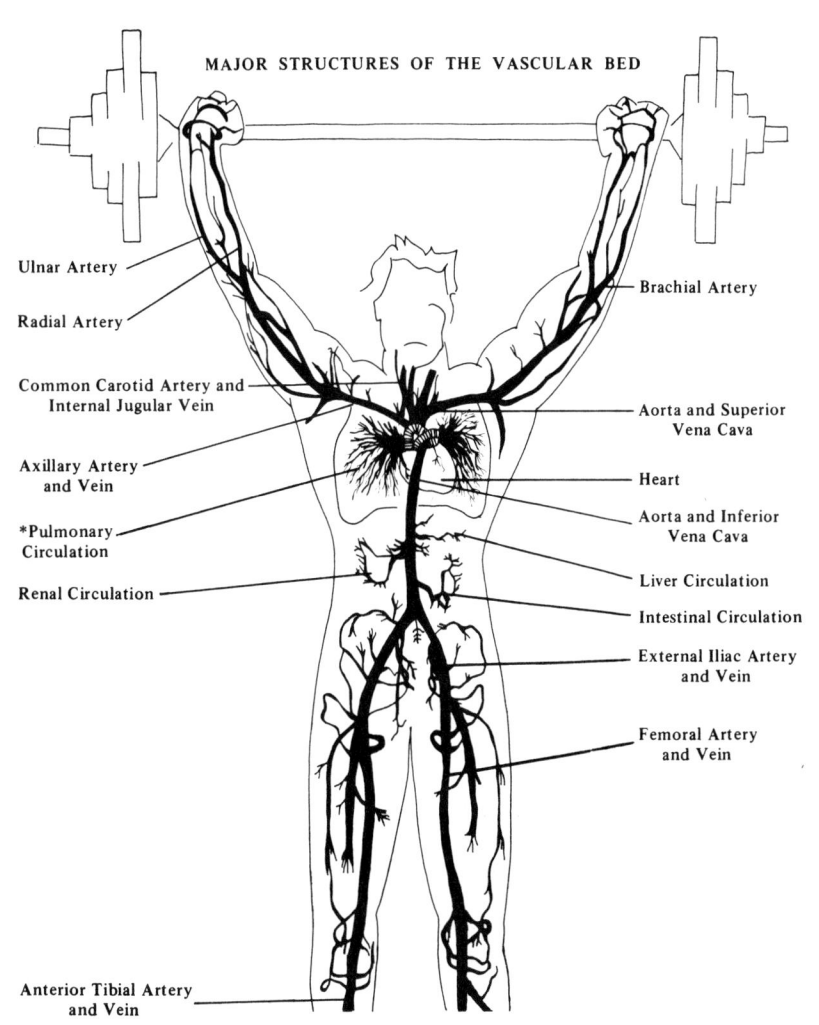

- Ulnar Artery
- Radial Artery
- Common Carotid Artery and Internal Jugular Vein
- Axillary Artery and Vein
- *Pulmonary Circulation
- Renal Circulation
- Brachial Artery
- Aorta and Superior Vena Cava
- Heart
- Aorta and Inferior Vena Cava
- Liver Circulation
- Intestinal Circulation
- External Iliac Artery and Vein
- Femoral Artery and Vein
- Anterior Tibial Artery and Vein

*Note: Function of Pulmonary Circulation		
Component	Description	Function
Pulmonary artery	Artery from the heart to the lungs	Brings blood with reduced oxygen and increased carbon dioxide and water to the lungs for diffusion through the capillary network for expiration.
Pulmonary veins	Veins from the lungs to the heart	Returns blood rich in oxygen to the heart for transportation to the tissues; exchange of gases between blood and body tissues is called internal respiration.

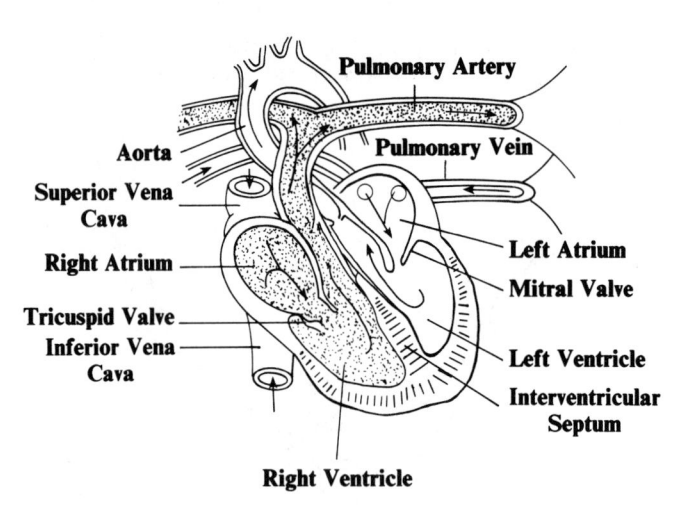

[Diagram of heart with labels: Aorta, Superior Vena Cava, Right Atrium, Tricuspid Valve, Inferior Vena Cava, Right Ventricle, Pulmonary Artery, Pulmonary Vein, Left Atrium, Mitral Valve, Left Ventricle, Interventricular Septum]

▨ **Deoxygenated Blood**
☐ **Oxygenated Blood**

Note: Function of Circulatory System (flow of nutritive fluids, waste materials and water)		
Component	Description	Function
Blood	About 12 pints of fluid tissue consisting of plasma (fluid) and blood cells (solid)	Carries nutrients to cells, removes cell wastes and water, carries oxygen to tissues, equalizes body temperature, distributes ductless gland secretions
Pulmonary circulation	Involves right side of heart, lung capillaries and pulmonary veins	Blood from body is pumped from the right ventricle through the pulmonary arteries to lungs; blood discharges carbon dioxide and water, picks up oxygen and returns to the left atrium through pulmonary veins
Systemic circulation	Left side of heart, aorta, arteries, capillaries and veins leading to venae cavae, plus several shorter circulations	Oxygenated blood pumped from left ventricle through the aorta to arteries and capillaries and returned through venules and veins to venae cavae, then to the right atrium
Coronary circulation	Aorta, coronary arteries and veins	Blood flows through the heart muscle, coronary arteries and veins; every heartbeat depends on free flow through these coronary vessels

THE MAJOR STRUCTURES OF THE RESPIRATORY SYSTEM

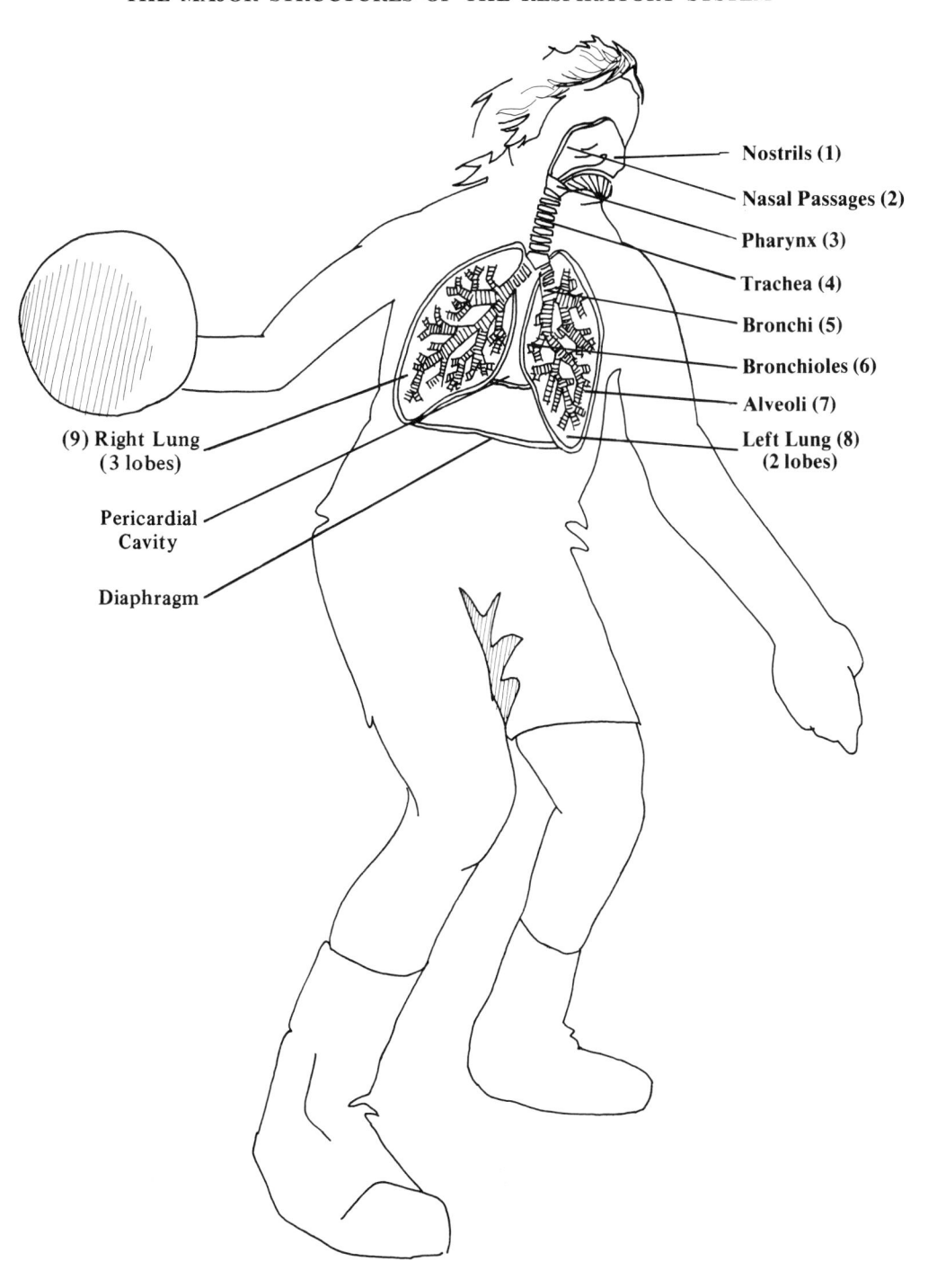

Nostrils (1)
Nasal Passages (2)
Pharynx (3)
Trachea (4)
Bronchi (5)
Bronchioles (6)
Alveoli (7)

(9) Right Lung
(3 lobes)

Left Lung (8)
(2 lobes)

Pericardial Cavity

Diaphragm

33

Function of the Respiratory System (Ventilation—External Respiration)		
Component	Description	Function
Nostrils (1)	Two nose openings divided by a wall called the septum	Contains hair for filtering impurities; air intake begins here and through the mouth
Nasal passages (2)	Joins nostrils to pharynx	Warms air, adds moisture on the way to pharynx
Pharynx (3)	Muscular throat cavity extends from nasal cavity to soft palate (uvula)	Common passageway for breathing and digestion; air passes to the trachea
Trachea (4)	Windpipe, a tube supported by horseshoe shaped rings of cartilage, closed by epiglottis (cartilaginous flap) during swallowing	Air passage to lungs lined with cilia in constant motion, carries impurities upward toward mouth as air descends to bronchi
Bronchi (5)	Trachea branches into two passages; each bronchus extends to one lung, subdivides into countless bronchial tubes	Air moves through bronchi into bronchioles inside the lungs
Bronchioles (6) Alveoli (7)	Countless subdivisions of bronchial tubes, ending in air sacs made up of protrusions called alveoli; each sac is surrounded by capillaries (tiny blood vessels)	Air sac and capillary walls are thin and moist, permit external respiration—the exchange of oxygen from air to blood with carbon dioxide and water from blood to air
Left lung (2 lobes) (8) right lung (3 lobes) (9)	Two organs composed of spongy tissue surrounded by a double membrane, consisting mainly of bronchioles with tiny air sacs, blood vessels and capillaries; total surface area about 2,000 square feet	Supply oxygen by way of the blood to millions of body cells having no direct access to oxygen; return waste gases and water vapor to the atmosphere

FUNCTION OF THE RESPIRATORY SYSTEM

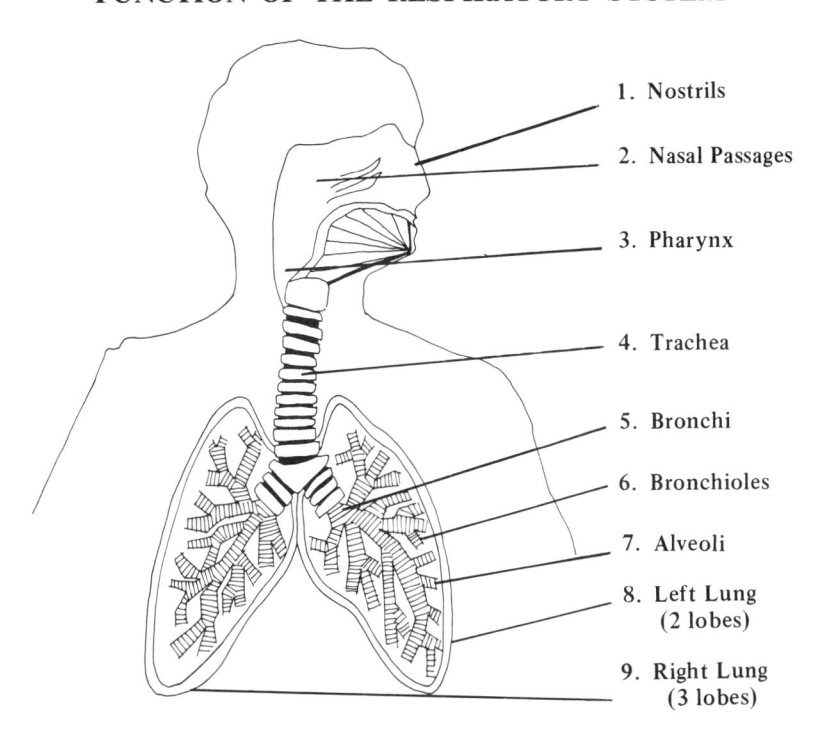

1. Nostrils
2. Nasal Passages
3. Pharynx
4. Trachea
5. Bronchi
6. Bronchioles
7. Alveoli
8. Left Lung (2 lobes)
9. Right Lung (3 lobes)

Cardio-Respiratory Function During Exercise

The fundamental action of the cardio-respiratory system during exercise is that of gas transport. These organs provide the equipment and power necessary to transport oxygen from the lungs, circulate it throughout the body, and assist in eliminating metabolic wastes.

During exercise the cardio-respiratory system adjusts to meet increased energy requirements. The total body blood flow (cardiac output) can increase enormously due primarily to an increase in heart rate and stroke volume. Blood flow to areas such as the kidneys and stomach which are not essential during exercise is decreased due to constriction of the arterioles. This, along with dilation of the arterioles in the working muscles, allows more oxygenated blood to be available to the muscles.

Aerobic/Anerobic Oxygen Utilization

During all forms of exercise, the increased demand for oxygen by the cells results in an increase in the depth and rate of breathing. The extent of this increased respiration rate depends upon the type, duration and intensity of exercise.

When oxygen utilization is equal to oxygen requirement, a "steady state" occurs in which the individual may persist in activity for extended periods of time. This is referred to as AEROBIC (with air) activity—exemplified in distance running.

When oxygen intake is unable to fulfill the energy requirement of intense exercise the anerobic energy systems supply the majority of energy. Exercise of this intensity is termed **ANEROBIC** (without air). Physical activity of this nature may continue for a short period of time, the extent depending upon ones anaerobic energy systems capacity and stress tolerance. The anaerobic energy system supplies energy for up to four minutes. Sprinting, in which one cannot maintain high levels of maximal work output for long time periods, exemplifies anaerobic activity.

Training Effects upon the Cardio-Respiratory System

Training effect can be defined as the positive physiological and psychological changes which can be produced as a result of involvement in physical activity. The extent of these positive effects are directly influenced by the nature, duration, intensity and frequency of the activity program. These aerobic training requirements are the necessary ingredients for assuring the production of cardio-respiratory training benefits. These four factors must be present in some form if changes in the aerobic energy pathways are to occur.

THE NATURE OF THE ACTIVITY and intensity of activity are inherently related since the type of motor activity selected determines the potential intensity. Participating in activities such as bowling and horseshoes limit or restrict intensity. Racquetball, cross-country skiing and jogging are capable of producing high levels of intensity.

INTENSITY OF EXERCISE dictates the degree of rise in resting heart rate. Exercise must be intense enough to raise the heart rate to target or threshold levels if training effects are to occur.

THE DURATION, length of time spent in continuous activity, should be a minimum of 12–15 minutes. The heart rate must increase to threshold levels and maintain this rate for a period of time (10–12 min.). The ideal duration of the activity is approximately 30 minutes per exercise bout. Research indicates that after 30 minutes of activity the law of diminishing return begins to take effect.

THE FREQUENCY OF TRAINING should occur a minimum of twice weekly and ideally every other day. This provides the body with adequate time for recovery. If one is concerned with high levels of competition or weight loss, increased duration and frequency would be appropriate once tolerance is developed.

Cardio-respiratory Training Affect Requirements

1. Nature of Activity—Determines potential to produce training effects.
2. Intensity—Heart Rate must raise to threshold levels.
3. Duration—Minimum of twelve–fifteen minutes per exercise bout.
4. Frequency—Exercise bouts should occur at least three times per week.

The changes which take place in the cardio-respiratory system resulting from training are extremely beneficial to the individual. The trained individual will experience:

1. lowered resting heart rate
2. lowered heart rate in response to submaximal exercise
3. increased resting stroke volume
4. increased maximal stroke volume
5. increased cardiac output
6. greater extraction of oxygen from arterial blood
7. increased static and dynamic lung volume
8. increased diffusing capacity at maximal work loads
9. increased blood volume
10. increased amount of hemoglobin
11. increased ability to tolerate lactic acid
12. increased aerobic and anaerobic capacity

The trained individual may experience:

1. increased number of coronary blood vessels
2. increased vessel size
3. increased efficiency of the heart
4. increased arterial oxygen content
5. increased clot dissolving capability
6. increased efficiency of peripheral blood distribution
7. increased efficiency of heart
8. increased thyroid function
9. increased growth hormone production
10. increased tolerance to stress
11. better living habits
12. decreased serum cholesterol levels
13. decreased arterial blood pressure
14. decreased over-reaction to hormones
15. decreased strain associated with psychic stress
16. decreased obesity

DEVELOPMENT OF CARDIO-RESPIRATORY CAPACITY

Examples of exercise used in developing C-R capacity are those which involve self-propulsion of the body for an extended period of time. The propulsion should be sufficiently severe and prolonged in order to ensure the adaptation of the circulatory and respiratory systems to the effort. Efficient forms of continuous exercise, since they can be reasonably well controlled, are running, jogging, and swimming. Distance, intensity and duration can be determined in accordance with the exercise tolerance of the individual. In addition, overload can be calculated and progression carefully planned. Other activities such as vigorous walking, rope skipping, skiing, and skating have similar values. Many sports requiring sustained running such as; soccer, basketball, handball and hockey have the potential to develop C.R.C. The deconditioned individual should exercise caution in sports participation so that the competitive element does not lead to overexertion.

Cardio-Respiratory Fitness and Active Living

Degenerative diseases such as obesity, loss of muscular tone, high blood pressure and arteriosclerosis are caused in part by lack of regular physical activity. These degenerative diseases are factors directly related to Coronary Heart Disease (CHD). This disease, which is the leading cause of death in the United States, kills over 700,000 people annually. It is estimated that over 6,000,000 Americans suffer from CHD.

A number of factors determine the degree of risk that each of us face in developing CHD. Included within the following list are factors in which we have little or no conscious influence, and others which we can directly control. Many of these factors are influenced by vigorous physical activity and diet depicted in the chart.

Cardiac Heart Disease

A. Lacking Conscious Control
1. Sex
2. Family History of Heart Disease
3. Elevated Uric Acid Levels
4. Lung Abnormalities
5. Cardiac Abnormalities

B. Influenced by Conscious Control
1. Blood Pressure
2. Obesity
3. Lipid Level
4. Behavioral Tendencies
5. Stress Adaptation

CARDIAC HEART DISEASE RISK FACTORS

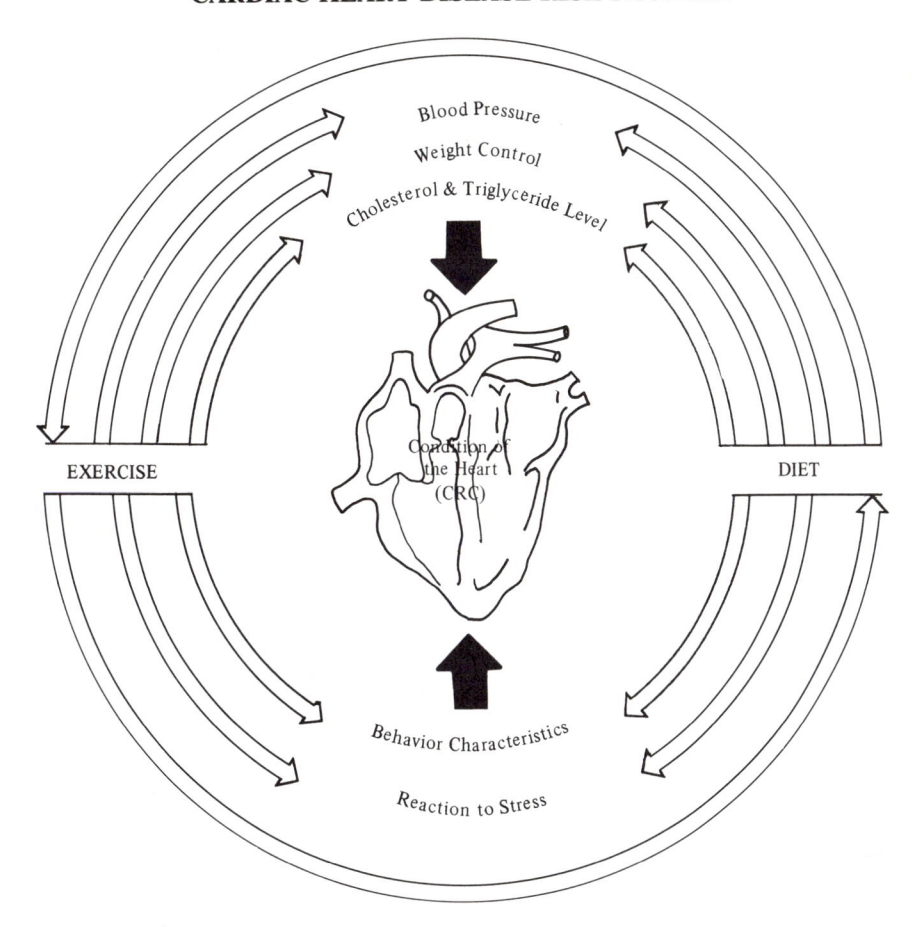

Blood Pressure
Weight Control
Cholesterol & Triglyceride Level

EXERCISE

Condition of the Heart (CRC)

DIET

Behavior Characteristics
Reaction to Stress

CORONARY HEART DISEASE

Coronary heart disease is just one form of cardiovascular disease. Other forms include high blood pressure (hypertension), stroke, rheumatic heart disease and congenital defects. Unlike many infectious diseases, it is difficult to identify the cause of coronary heart disease since a number of factors influence its development. In addition, it is often difficult to discover its presence.

Scientists have carefully investigated the manner in which our way of life is related to heart disease. The great increase in coronary heart disease since the year 1900 may be related to the drastic changes in lifestyles that have occurred in our culture. Our lives have become more urban and highly mechanized. We ride elevators, escalators, buses and automobiles rather than walk. We subject ourselves to high levels of stress, smoke more cigarettes and engage in less physical activity. We eat foods that are engorged with calories, starch, sugar, saturated fats, artificial flavorings and coloring, and are processed with chemical preservatives.

Physicians and medical researchers generally agree that stress, high blood pressure, smoking, elevated cholesterol levels and obesity are major risk factors. Risk is a statistical expression of probability, and is not to be confused with cause. Each additional risk factor to which a person is exposed seems to increase their likelihood of developing coronary heart disease. The major risk factors may occur singly, but more often are found in some multiple form. Fortunately, risk of coronary heart disease can be reduced by medical supervision or eliminated by a change in lifestyle.

The risk factors associated with increased incidence of coronary heart disease are complex and interrelated:

Blood Fat Pattern may show types of altered proportions of blood fats. One in particular is characterized by raised cholesterol levels in the blood. Other types are characterized by elevations in blood fats, such as triglyceride. Altered blood fat patterns can indicate risk.

Diet: The role of diet in coronary heart disease is still not completely understood. It is interesting to note the profound relationship of diet and three of the major risk factors; obesity, cholesterol and triglyceride levels, and blood pressure. A patient diagnosed as suffering from coronary heart disease will usually be placed on a strict diet resulting in control of these factors.

Several approaches are often undertaken to lower an individual's risk profile through diet. These may include reduction in saturated fatty acids, cholesterol, calories, salt, refined sugar and/or an increase in polyunsaturated fatty acids and fiber.

Obesity: When more calories are consumed than are burned during physical activity, the additional calories are stored as fat, (adipose tissue), and a person may become overweight or obese. Obesity is a coronary heart disease risk factor and is often associated with diabetes, high blood pressure, raised blood cholesterol, and elevated blood triglycerides. Frequently, decreasing caloric intake to attain desirable body weight tends to normalize blood fat patterns and decrease high blood pressure.

Exercise: Becoming a sedentary person increases the danger of coronary heart disease as inactivity tends to increase body weight. Physical activity is an important aspect of a weight control program. In addition, physical activity improves blood circulation throughout the entire body and in the coronary arteries in the heart. Blood cholesterol and triglycerides both tend to be lowered and the tendency to form blood clots is reduced through exercise.

The interdependence of a nutritionally-balanced diet, sensible weight control, regular exercise and consultation with physicians concerning special problems should be recognized as the wisest course to follow on the road to reducing susceptibility to coronary heart disease.

The evidence accumulated through research demonstrates the positive effects activity and conditioning have on cardio-respiratory capacity. While exercise does not affect heredity, sex and structural abnormalities, it has a pronounced positive influence on body weight, blood pressure, obesity, blood, lipid levels and hopefully health habits. While these areas function with others in cause and effect of cardiac heart disease, we are able to consciously control the majority of factors as preventative measures. We can stop smoking, follow a healthy diet, control body weight, improve cardio-respiratory condition and limit stressful life-styles. In short, it is possible that in our lifetime we can see coronary heart disease diminished as a critical health problem if we have the will to structure our life-styles based on intelligence and determination.

Selected References

Astrand, P. O. and Rodahl, K. *Textbook of Work Physiology* (2nd Ed.) New York: McGraw-Hill, 1977.

Baldwin, K. M., Fitts, R. H., Booth, F. W., Wider, W. W. and Holloszy, J. O. *Depletion of Muscle and Liver Glycogen during Exercise.* Pflugers Archives. 1975, 354, 203–212.

Holloszy, J. Biochemical adaptation of exercise: Aerobic Metabolism. In J. Wilmore (Ed.) *Exercise and Sport Sciences Reviews.* New York: Academic Press. 1973.

Saltin, B. and Astrand, P. O. Maximal oxygen uptake in athletics. *Journal of Applied Physiology,* 1967, 23, 353–358.

Saltin, B. and Karlsson, J. In B. Pernow and B. Saltin (Eds.), *Muscle Metabolism During Exercise.* New York: Planum, 1971.

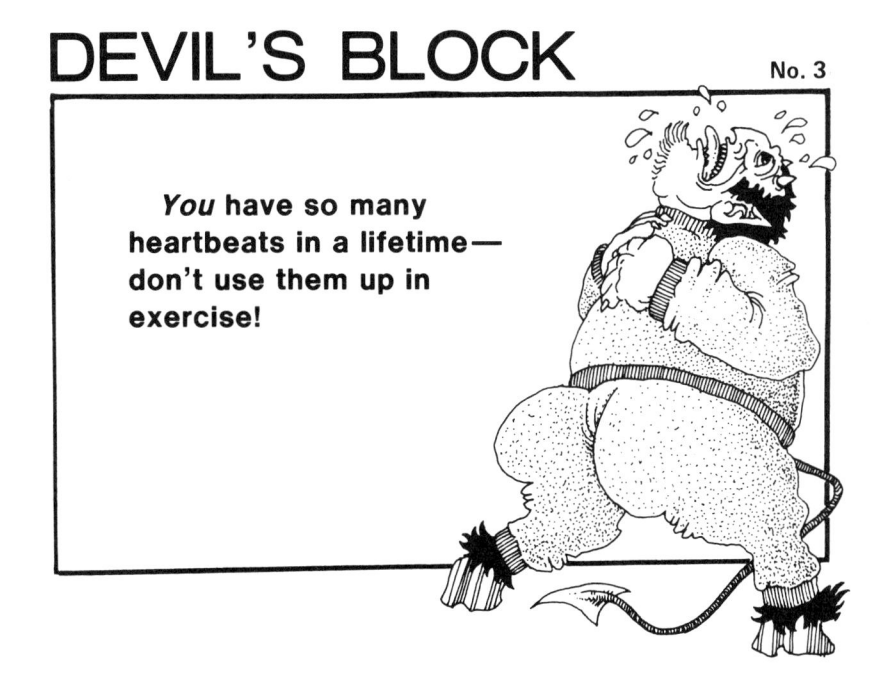

DEVIL'S BLOCK No. 3

You have so many heartbeats in a lifetime— don't use them up in exercise!

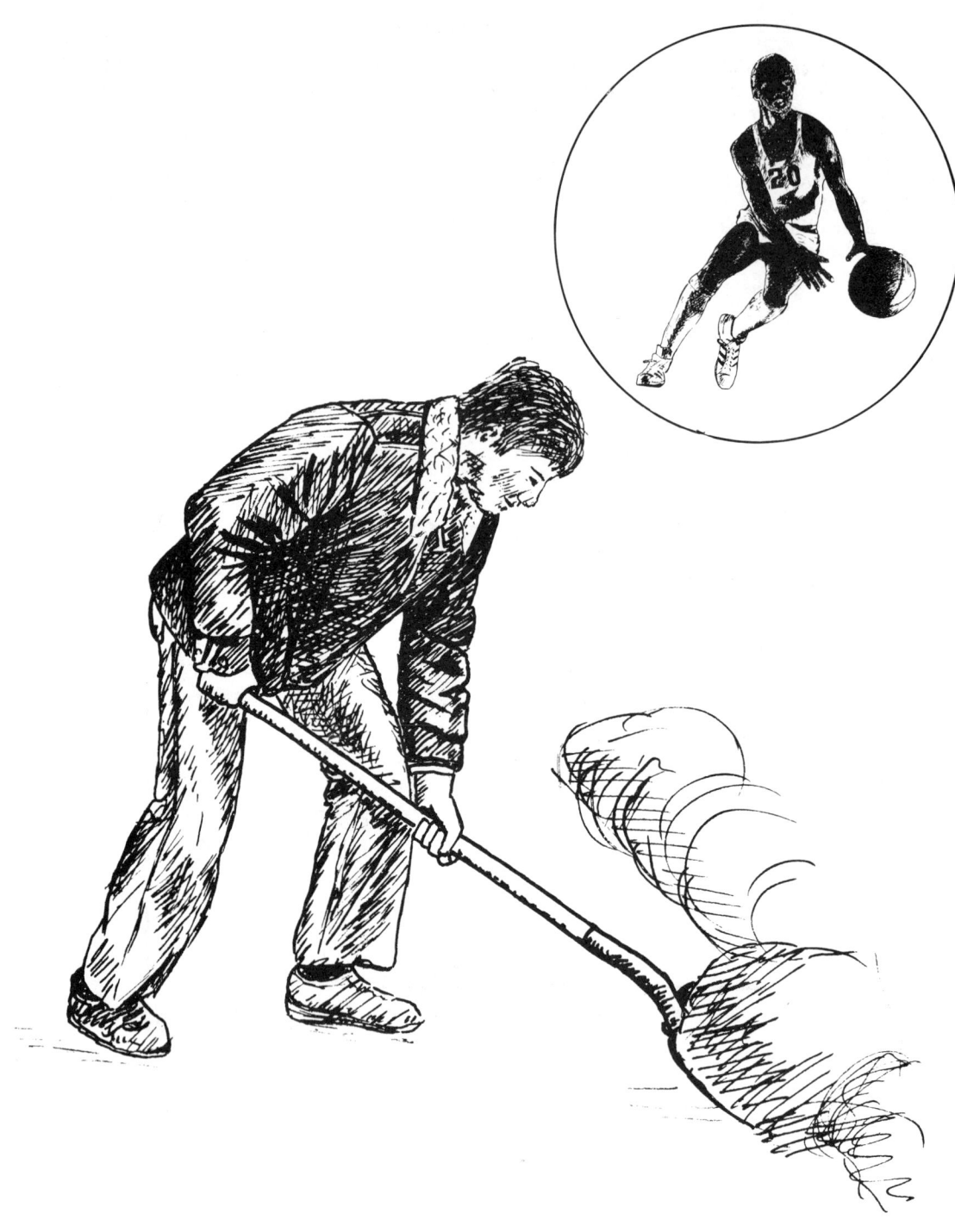

CARDIO-RESPIRATORY CAPACITY

PERSONAL APPRAISAL 3
Cardio-Respiratory Capacity

Physical activity may have a significant and positive affect upon the physiological condition of the heart, lungs and circulatory system. From a purely health-related standpoint, the relationship of cardio-respiratory capacity (CRC), body weight and diet to degenerative disease of the heart and circulatory system seem crucial. Although regular exercise, and its positive influence on CRC, is but one of several factors that may help prevent degenerative heart disease, it is of vital importance because of its favorable influence upon body weight and stress tolerance.

A thorough evaluation of one's present state of cardio-respiratory capacity will provide us with valuable information that may shed light on our potential to develop degenerative heart disease. It will also provide us with a starting point that will allow us to establish realistic goals and construct a meaningful and sequential conditioning program.

Equipment and Facilities

A. 440-Yard Track

B. Stopwatch

C. 18" Bench

D. Area for Nonlocomotor Exercise and 60-Yard Dash

Procedures

A. *6 minute walk-run for distance*—This has become an accepted test of cardio-respiratory capacity. It correlates closely with oxygen uptake as measured in the laboratory. This is also considered a measure of aerobic capacity.

  1. Using a 440-yard track, walk-run for the greatest possible distance within 6 minutes. Record your score to the nearest eighth of a lap.

_____ Distance Covered

B. *Exercise intensity and heart rate*—With this experiment, we are able to discover how different types and intensities of exercise affect heart rate. In order for exercise to be of value to the cardio-respiratory system, the heart rate must reach the "Threshold of Training" (minimum level that will produce the training affect). For most of us, a minimum heart rate of 145 will produce adequate results. A more accurate measure of the threshold is found in number 3 below. Implications of CRC may also be derived from this test.

1. Find the carotid pulse by placing the index and middle fingers of the hand slightly above and alongside the thyroid cartilage. With slight pressure from the fingertips, you should be able to feel the pulse.

2. Compute your resting heart rate—while seated and fully rested, take a ten second carotid pulse reading, multiply by six and record your results.

_____ Resting Heart Rate

3. Compute your personal threshold of training level by subtracting your age from 220. This is your predicted maximal heart rate. Subtract your resting heart rate from the predicted maximum rate. Compute 60 percent of this difference and add it to your resting rate. This will be the pulse rate necessary to bring adequate CRC gains.

_____ Threshold Heart Rate

4. Walk for one minute at a medium speed. Sit, and within ten seconds of completion of exercise, take a ten-second carotid pulse reading. Multiply this by six and record under results. Rest for one minute before initiating next exercise.

_____ Heart Rate After Walking

5. Walk up a flight of stairs, at least fifteen steps. Measure and record pulse rate. Rest for one minute.

_____ Heart Rate After Walk-Up

6. Run in place for one minute. As before, measure and record pulse rate. Rest for one minute before next exercise.

_____ Heart Rate After Running

7. "Jumping Jack"—Jump to side stride, arms sideward and upward—return to starting position. In cadence for thirty seconds. Measure and record pulse rate. Rest for one minute.

_____ Heart Rate After "Jumping Jack"

8. "Curlups"—Supine position—draw knees up and curl upper body to sitting position and return. Repeat for 30 seconds. Measure and record pulse rate. Rest for one minute.

_____ Heart Rate After "Curlups"

9. Perform the four-count burpee (squat, hands on ground, extend legs, recover legs and stand) for one minute to instructor's cadence. Measure and record pulse rate as before. Rest for one minute before next exercise.

_____ Heart Rate After Burpee

10. Sprint at full speed a distance of 60 yards. Measure and record pulse rate.

_____ Heart Rate After Sprint

C. *Modified Step Test*—The step test is an accepted measure of post-exercise recovery time. The ability to recover is related to CRC.
  1. Work with a partner; one person recording, while the other is being tested.
  2. Find and record the resting heart rate for one minute.

_____ Resting Heart Rate

  3. Use an 18 inch bench or step.
  4. Using a four-count cadence, step up on the bench with either foot on the count of one. Be sure that the foot is placed completely on the bench. Bring the other foot up on the bench on the count of two so that the knees are straight. Step down with the foot placed on the bench first on the count of three, and bring the other foot down on four. This four-count pace should occur every two seconds.
  5. For a maximum of ten seconds, practice stepping up and down on the bench until the correct rhythm is established.
  6. Perform the test for a period of three minutes. Upon completion, sit and immediately count heart rate for ten seconds, multiply by six and record.

_____ Heart Rate After Exercise

  7. Rest for one minute and repeat the count and recording of heart rate as above.

_____ Heart Rate After 1½ Minutes

  8. Repeat counting and recording the heart rate after one minute's rest two more additional times.

_____ Heart Rate After 3 Minutes

_____ Heart Rate After 4½ Minutes

  9. Find difference between your resting heart rate and heart rate three minutes after exercise.

_____ Difference

Compare the difference of your resting heart rate and heart rate three minutes after exercise with the difference of *ten* other people.

1. _____

2. _____

3. _____

4. _____

5. _____

6. _____

7. _____

8. _____

9. _____

10. _____

Average Difference _____ .

EVALUATION REPORT
Personal Appraisal No. 3

Name _____

Date _____

Lifetime Participation

I. *Laboratory Title:* Cardio-Respiratory Capacity

II. *Objective:*

III. *Results:*

A. *6 minute walk-run*—Distance Traveled _____

"Women are just the same as men except for here and there and every now and then." This is one example of an "every now and then."

Men	Scale	Women
Laps		**Laps**
4¼	Excellent	3¾
3¾	Very good	3¼
3¼	Good	2¾
2¾	Fair	2¼
2¼	Poor	1¾
Less 2¼	Extreme deconditioned	Less 1¾

Threshold of Training

1. 220 − Age = Adjusted Maximal Heart Rate _____ − Resting Heart Rate ____

2. Subtract Resting Heart Rate from #1   _____

3. 60% of Difference of #2   _____

4. Add Resting Heart Rate to #3   _____ = Threshold

B. *Exercise Intensity and Pulse Rate*

Data

Resting Heart Rate _____

One Minute Walking Heart Rate _____

Fifteen Step Climb _____

One Minute Run in Place Heart Rate _____

Thirty Second—Jumping Jack _____

Thirty Second—Curlups _____

One Minute Four-Count Burpee Heart Rate _____

60-Yard Dash Heart Rate _____

Compare the above heart rates with others.

C. *Recovery Time—Three Minute Modified Step Test*

Data

Heart Rate

1. Resting _____

2. Immediately After Exercise _____

3. 1½ Minutes After Exercise _____

4. Three Minutes After Exercise _____

5. 4½ Minutes After Exercise _____

6. Difference between #1 and #4 _____

7. Average of the comparison made with 10 other people _____

8. Difference between #6 (your score) and #7 (ave. of 10 others) _____

IV. *Analysis:*

   1. What insights have you gained in taking this personal appraisal?

   2. Compare the recovery of your heart rate in Text C with the recovery of ten other people of the same sex.

   3. Provide the reasons for your state of cardiovascular endurance.

   4. Is the state of your cardio-respiratory endurance important to you at this time of your life? Explain!

V. *Implications:*

    1. Discuss the implications of the results of test 2 and 3.

    2. What events or situations would have to occur for you to be stimulated to improve the state of your cardio-respiratory endurance?

    3. Describe the activities that you would be interested in participating in that would result in your improved cardio-respiratory endurance.

4
FLEXIBILITY

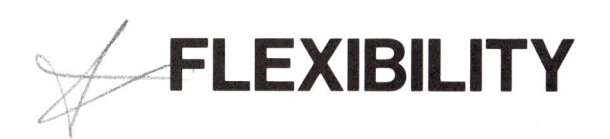

Flexibility can be defined as the range of motion of the articulations. The importance of freedom of joint movement becomes apparent when we view the prevalence of health problems of the articulation system, such as low back pain, postural deviations, and arthritis. These infirmities affect vast numbers of Americans and can often be directly related to a loss or limit of flexibility.

Joint flexibility is determined by a variety of anatomical factors. Bone structure and ligaments determine range of motion as well as the connective tissue of tendons and muscle. Changes in tendon and muscle tissue length can be brought about through stretching. Muscles and tendons adapt in length according to their pattern of use. If muscles function with a limited range of motion, they tend to shorten with accompanying loss of flexibility. Injuries, such as strains, sprains and fractures, also result in a loss in range of motion.

When body articulations are supple, a great amount of flexibility is available. Conversely, when these structures lose their ability to stretch, flexibility decreases and there is increased potential for the onset of degenerative joint diseases.

Some of the possible causes of loss of flexibility are:

1. injured or diseased joint surfaces—many types of arthritis restrict, and in some cases, eliminate movement.
2. shortened muscles and tendons—this condition usually results from poor daily posture and body mechanics. An example would be sleeping on one's stomach which is a poor sleeping posture and will often result in pain and shortened muscles in the region of the lower back.
3. damaged ligaments—the ligaments are bands of connective tissue that function in providing joint stability and actually hold the joint together. When these structures become damaged, the resulting pain limits the use and flexibility of the joint.
4. calcification—severe strain on joints may result in the production of calcium and bursa deposits which, because of their position in the joint, cause pain and restrict movement.
5. pain—the pain which accompanies many joint diseses and injuries becomes a major problem in that the resulting lack of use caused by the pain often results in decreased flexibility which can have a negative affect on the underlying problem.
6. muscle boundness—the use of this term has been misleading. If the antagonist or opposing muscle or group of muscles is developed along with the agonist muscles, flexibility is not affected. It is only when the agonist is developed with no attention given to the antagonist that unbalanced development, along with a loss of flexibility occurs.
7. Through disuse—when our pattern of living results in discontinued stretching of muscles and tendons, loss of flexibility will occur.

PRINCIPLES OF FLEXIBILITY

Flexibility can be produced primarily by stretching the muscles and tendons. The term "stretch" implies elongation, a linear deformation in the direction of increased length. Stretching refers to the process of elongation. Stretch is not present without an increase in length beyond the resting state of the structure. Any movement to this point would be comparable to merely reducing slack.

There are two types of stretch:

1. Elastic Stretch—Represents spring-like behavior: Any elongation by tensile loading is recovered following removal of the load. It is therefore described as temporary recoverable elongation.
2. Plastic stretch—refers to putty-like behavior: in which the elongation produced by tensile stress remains even when the stress is removed. This is decribed as non-recoverable or permanent elongation. We should strive for plastic stretch in our flexibility program.

The relative degree of elastic and plastic deformation will vary widely depending upon the methods and the conditions under which stretching is performed. The principle factors involved in stretching are: amount of force; duration of force; and tissue temperature.

Stretching, is the primary method of increasing flexibility. Stretching is usually accomplished in one of two methods:

1. Static stretching—A low force stretching method, in which stretching movements occur slowly and are held for a period of time.
2. Ballistic stretching—High force stretching, in which the stretching movements occur in short rather violent bursts.

Static Sretching exercises, with slow rhythmical and sustained movements, are recommended as the most efficient means of increasing flexibility. The portion of tissue lengthening that remains, is greater, once the tensile stress is removed through this low-force, long duration method. Research indicates that ballistic stretching may produce the opposite result of those desired since the violent stretch may result in a reflex contraction which causes the muscle to shorten. Ballistic stretching does not enhance plastic deformation. It may also weaken muscle tissue and it can possibly cause muscle rupture. Any activity in which stretch is applied slowly and maintained steadily will allow muscles and tendons to relax and permit themselves to become elongated. Using this technique of stretching for even brief periods of each day will produce increased flexibility in a short time.

Flexibility is an ongoing and continuous variable. This implies that movement, which increases or maintains flexibility, should be practiced regularly throughout life. The result of stretching is long-lasting yet will gradually decrease if flexibility exercise is discontinued.

It is unnecessary in terms of daily living to develop levels of flexibility such as those of gymnasts and dancers. It is important that we are able to maintain degrees of suppleness that will allow us to resist the degenerative health problems associated with loss of flexibility and permit us to function efficiently in our daily lives.

"PREVENTION" OF INJURY THROUGH FLEXIBILITY

Increasing and maintaining flexibility is important in the prevention of injury, especially in reducing the great number of nuisance injuries referred to as mucular strain. Disguised under the term, "pull," these injuries often constitute a serious and sometimes painful athletic injury.

For years, sports medicine experts have expressed different opinions concerning the causes of this type of injury. It is generrlly agreed that fatigue, incorrect posture, muscular imbalance, poor flexibility, and overstretching are the primary causes leading to such strains. However, despite the fact that these causative factors are known and accepted, there still remains for the "sports medicine team," the physicians, athletic trainer and coach, the responsibility of preventing injuries of this type by stressing the importance of flexibility through proper static movements.

Hypotheses

If you increase the range of motion in a joint, and you should be confronted with a situation which requires explosive movement or extreme extention or flexion, injury is prevented since the articulation can now accept the additional stress. This situation can occur throughout all activity. Give yourself this "preventive" edge by striving for full range or motion in all the articulations in the body.

Selected References

Clark, H. H. (Ed.): Joint and body range of movement. In *Physical Fitness Research Digest.* Washington, D.C., Presidents Council on Physical Fitness and Sports, Series 5, No. 4. 1975.

Holland, G.: The physiology of flexibility: A review of the literature. *Kinesiology Review,* 1968, pp. 49–62.

Holt, L. E.: *Scientific stretching for sport.* Halifax, Nova Scotia, Canada, Sport Research Ltd., 1976.

Johns, R., and Wright, V.: Relative importance of various tissues in joint stiffness. *J. Appl. Physiology.,* 17: 824–828, 1962.

Mathews, D.: *Measurement in Physical Education.* 4th Ed. Philadelphia, W. B. Saunders Co., 1973.

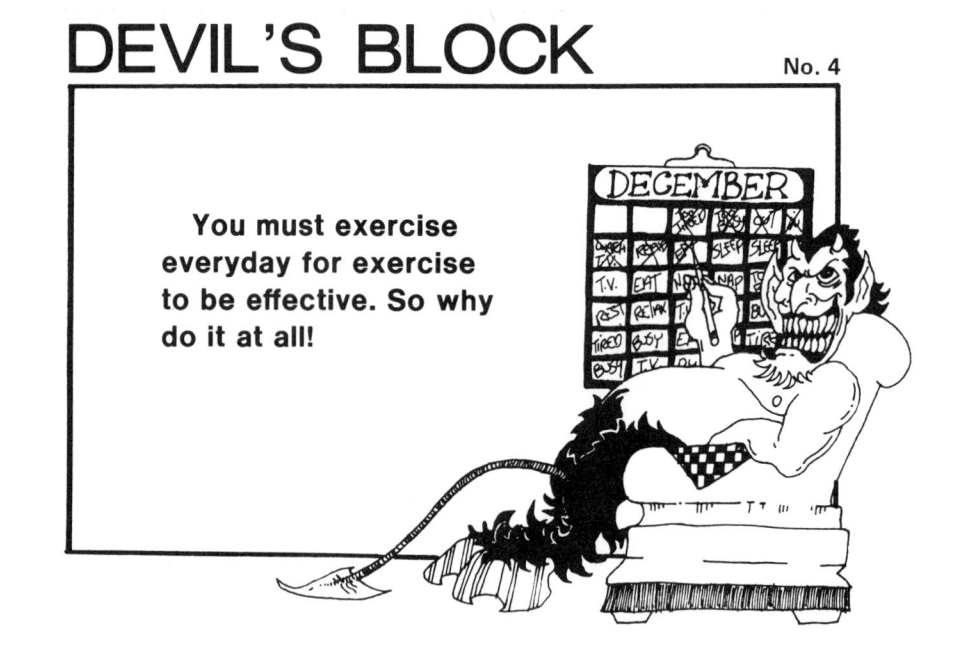

DEVIL'S BLOCK No. 4

You must exercise everyday for exercise to be effective. So why do it at all!

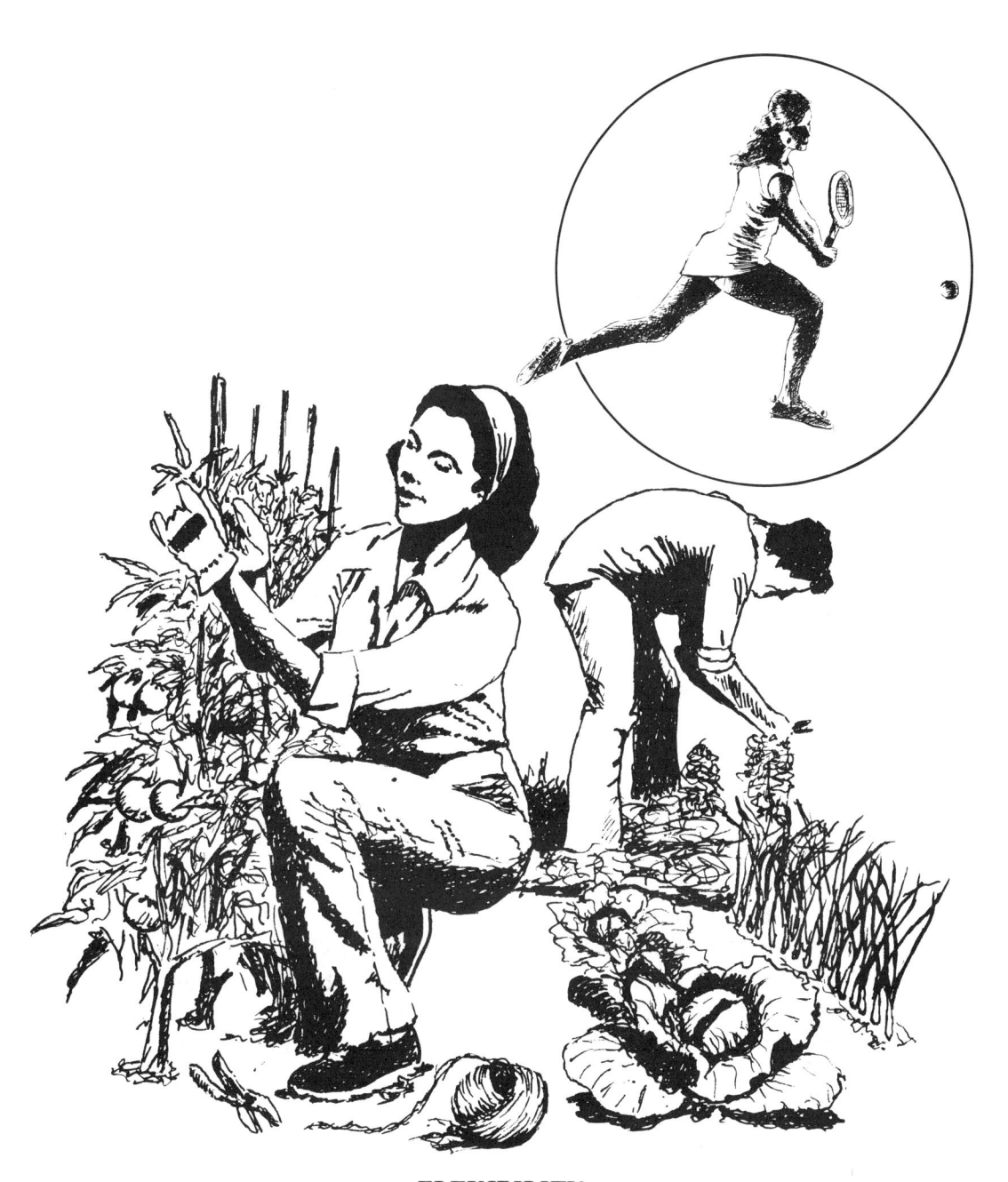

FLEXIBILITY

PERSONAL APPRAISAL NO. 4
Flexibility

This apraisal functions both as an introduction to basic flexibility movements and in evaluating one's present state of flexibility. Are you a flexible person? This is a difficult question to answer since flexibility is peculiar to individual articulations. A person could have extreme ranges of motion in various joints and little flexibility in others.

There are relatively few individuals who are flexible in all articulations of the body. The concept of overall body flexibility is a standard we should all strive to achieve.

There are two primary reasons for deep concern about the maintenance of flexibility. Flexibility is a significant factor in the prevention of common muscle and tendon injuries. In addition, it can increase the performance potential of an athlete by providing a greater range of motion in the application of muscular strength.

Equipment and Facilities

    A. Exercise mat is advisable

    B. Yardstick

    C. Box or Bench—12" High
                            8" Wide
                            18" Long

Procedures

Complete this appraisal with the assistance of a partner.

    A. Hamstring and lower back flexibility test.

        1. Utilize a box or bench with a front side approximately 12–18" in height. Starting at the front edge mark off in half inch gradations 0–14 inches.

        2. Sit with both feet placed against the front side of the box, keeping the knees locked. Stretch slowly from the waist extending the arms forward as far as possible.

        3. Your partner will note and record the furthest point reached with the fingertips, to the nearest 1/2".

    B. General flexibility test

        1. Attempt to perform each of the test items. The movement should be gradual and smooth, and should be discontinued upon the onset of pain.

        2. Follow the brief description and illustration of each test item. All movements must be complete with a full range of motion. Record either pass or fail on each test.

Flexibility Test Items

Test Item	Description	Illustration	Pass	Fail
1. *Front Bend*	Standing position—clenched fist—bend forward and touch knuckles to floor—keeping knees locked.			
2. *Side Twist*	Standing position—feet shoulder width apart—fingers interlocked behind neck—flex forward at waist with knees locked—touch left elbow to right knee—then touch right elbow to left knee.			
3. *Tailor Sit*	Sitting position—soles of feet drawn up together—place hands on knees and push until knees touch the floor.			
4. *Front Curl*	Sitting position—interlocked behind head—curl forward with knees locked—touch head to knees.			
5. *Lotus Sit (Half) Right*	Sitting position—legs extended—lift and place the heel of the right foot on top of the left thigh, draw into midsection. Push right knee down 4″ from floor.			
6. *Lotus Sit (Half) Left*	Sitting position—same as above—but lift and place the heel of the left foot on top of the right thigh.			
7. *Swaying Palm*	Kneeling position—toes back—lean backward until head touches floor.			
8. *Criss-Cross (with partner)*	Standing position—arms extended to side with elbows locked and palms forward—from behind, partner grasps both wrists and stretches arms back to a parallel position (posture must be erect throughout).			

9. *Jackknife*—Lying on back (supine position) keeping knees locked draw legs up and over until feet touch floor.

10. *Arch*—Lying on stomach (prone position) hands behind neck—raise upper body until chin is 18″ from floor.

11. *Hammerlock (right hand)*—Standing position—reach behind the back with the left hand, palm facing outward, reach over the right shoulder with the right arm, extend the right hand toward the left hand. Attempt to touch fingers of both hands.

12. *Hammerlock (left hand)*—Reverse the directions for "hammerlock (right hand)."

13. *Cobra*—Prone position—place hands on floor to the side of shoulders. Extend arms, raising upper body and head in a posterior direction. Flex at the knee joint and attempt to touch the back of the head with the toes.

14. *Periscope (right leg)*—Sitting position—legs extended. Grab the right ankle with both hands, lean back, pulling the right leg up into a vertical position. Both knees are locked, left leg remaining on floor. Both legs form an "L" shape at completion.

15. *Periscope (left leg)*—Reverse the directions for "periscope (right leg)."

EVALUATION REPORT
Personal Appraisal No. 4

Name _____

Date _____

Lifetime Participation

  I. *Title:* Flexibility

 II. *Objective:*

III. *Results:*

    A. Hamstring and Lower Back Flexibility Test

Rating:	Hamstring and Lower Back	
Score	Category	
7.6–+	Excellent	1
5.6–7.5	Above average	2
3.6–5.5	Average	3
2.6–3.5	Below averge	4
Under–1.5	Poor	5

    B. General Flexibility Test:

      1. Circle Test Items Passed:

        1 2 3 4 5 6 7 8 9 10 11 12 13 14 15

      2. No. of Test Items Passed _____ × 2 = Flexibility Score _____

Category

1. Total Flexibility	—	26–30
2. Above Average	—	20–24
3. Average	—	14–18
4. Below Average	—	8–12
5. Poor	—	0–6

IV. *Analysis:*

    1. In your opinion, how are the results of this personal appraisal significant? Explain.

    2. List the test items passed on the General Flexibility Test:

    3. List the test items failed. Analyze the reasons for failure.

    4. In considering all the test items, how would you rate your overall flexibility. Explain!

    5. Describe activities that you presently engage in which would be enhanced by increased flexibility:

V. *Implications:*

    1. What program do you intend to follow to increase and maintain flexibility?

    2. Decribe the manner in which adequate levels of flexibility may be significant during your life.

5

MUSCULAR STRENGTH

Nearly all body movement occurs as a result of muscular contraction or relaxation. Conscious movement occurs as skeletal or voluntary muscle contracts, shortens and exerts tension on the skeletal system. This tension results in the activation of a system of levers which pull body parts such as the lower arm; hence movement. Skeletal muscles are composed of bundles of individual fibers each wrapped in a sheath of connective tissue. A motor neuron (nerve) enters the muscle and extends through the fibers ending in the area it will service. It branches from a few, to thousands of extensions which end on the plates attached to each individual fiber. An electrical impulse travels the length of the neuron causing a chemical change in the muscle fibers, resulting in a shortening of the fiber. This neuron, along with all of its innervated fibers, is called a motor unit. When many motor units are activated and the frequency of neuron discharge is high (from 5–50 impulses per second), a strong muscular contraction results.

Muscular Function During Exercise

Since muscle tissue is capable of exerting more force than can be ordinarily called upon, muscular strength can be referred to as maximal voluntary strength. In a maximal voluntary contraction, maximal contractile potential may never be reached. Research has demonstrated that electrical stimulation, hypnosis, drugs, and situations of fear or surprise are capable of eliciting muscle contraction of greater tension than those of maximal voluntary efforts.

Maximal voluntary strength can be defined as the ability to consciously exert maximum muscular tension such as an individual pressing the heaviest possible resistance on a barbell. Some of the important principles related to muscular strength are listed below.

1. Muscular strength is directly proportional to a muscle's cross-sectional area (girth).
2. A stretched muscle is capable of exerting greater force.
3. Muscle enlargement (hypertrophy) resulting from strength training is caused by an increase in the diameter of muscle fiber and development of connective tissue.
4. Strength training is the product of muscular tension and to a great extent repetitive movements.
5. Concentric contraction occurs when muscle fibers shorten in performing work. Most strength training involves programs which utilize this type of contraction.
6. Eccentric contractions occur when muscle fibers lengthen in producing work. It has been demonstrated that these types of contractions also promote strength increases.
7. Voluntary isotonic and isometric contraction produce increased strength.

8. Isotonic contractions occur when muscle contracts, angle of joints change, and body parts move.
9. Isometric contractions occur when muscle contracts, joint angles remain unchanged, and no movement of body parts results.

Isometric contraction does not seem to stimulate strength gains as efficiently as isotonic contractions. This may in part be due to the low motivation which may be found in isometric workouts due to the difficulty in perceiving the levels of work and force applied.

The challenge resulting from observing a resistance move is greater than in an isometric effort in which no observable work is accomplished.

A recently publicized principle of strength training termed "isokenetics" involves maximum resistance over a complete range of motion. This system has demonstrated impressive gains in strength in relatively short periods of time. Isokenetics equipment utilize hydrolic and electronic systems which change resistance throughout each movement of an exercise.

Principles of Muscular Strength Development

The development of muscular strength is based upon utilization of the *overload* principle. This concept implies that strength is the product of work accomplished at higher than normal levels. With the overload principle in operation, the following training effects along with a corresponding increase in strength will occur:

1. Hypertrophy or increased muscular size
2. Changes in motor pathways
3. Reduction of central nervous system inhibitions
4. Increase in connective tissue

Progressive resistance exercise has been universally recognized as the most appropriate means of eliciting training effects and building muscular strength and endurance. Experts throughout the world have adopted weight training as the most efficient method of producing rapid and highly significant strength gains. During weight training sessions the intensity of exercise can be regulated through careful adjustment of the amount of resistance, number of repetitions and sets, speed of movement, and the reduction of rest periods between bouts of exercise. Exercises can be designed to include all of the major muscle groups, correct muscular imbalance and improve strength related to the skill movements of virtually all sports. Circuit training can be utilized to bring forth cardio-respiratory endurance as well as gains in muscular strength. Progressive resistance exercise can provide an ideal means of producing increased strength and endurance, improved body tone and symmetry, additional flexibility and a heightened sense of health and vitality.

Women and Muscular Strength

Traditionally women have shied away from using strength developing techniques for fear of building bulging and defined muscle. This phenomena has had three unfortunate results. First many women simply choose to refrain from participation in physical activity. Secondly, many women have been unsuccessful in developing basic sports skills in activities requiring muscular strength and endurance such as track, racquet ball and gymnastics. Finally, this fear of massive muscular development has caused many fine women athletes to fall short of realizing their potential.

Research indicates that women who participate in strength building activities will develop gains in strength that are similar to men without experiencing the same level of hypertrophy. This is the result of hormonal and fat percentage differences in men and women. Women typically possess lower levels of testosterone a hormone that stimulates muscle development along with a greater percentage of subcutaneous fat. These two factors imply that women may place a great amount of emphasis on strength training and the resulting increase in muscular tonus without concern for developing highly defined muscular mass.

During the past few years we have observed the rise of competition among women "body builders" who have been able to develop mass and definition in their skeletal muscles. This may be the result of women who fall into the less than one percent possessing a high testosterone level, becoming involved in body building. In addition, some women have chosen to use steroids to help induce the condition of muscle hypertrophy. These factors have no bearing on women who embark upon a body shaping program for "aesthetic appearance" or strength building programs for fitness and sports conditioning.

Muscular Strength in Daily Living

Muscular contraction functions in some part of the human organism each moment of life. This shortening of muscle occurs in cardiac tissue which forces blood from the heart to the body's tissues, or in smooth muscle in the small intestine helping move foodstuffs through the alimentary tract, or skeletal muscle allowing conscious movement. The condition of muscle tissue determines to a great extent the degree of efficiency of human movement. Conditioned muscle permits us to function in our daily living with ease and comfort.

However, for most of us, great strength need not be a priority in our daily living. Some individuals such as professional athletes, movers and construction workers may require high levels of muscular strength.

Acceptable levels of strength will permit us to accomplish daily tasks involving work such as moving a loaded wheelbarrow or picking up a case of canned goods without experiencing fatigue or injury. It will also enable us to meet many emergencies in which strength may be required. In short, acceptable levels of muscular strength will assist us in making our daily lives less fatiguing and more enjoyable.

Selected References

Barnard, R., Edgerton, V., and Peter, J. Effects of exercise on skeletal muscle. I. Biochemical and histochemical properties. *Journal of Applied Physiology.* 1970, 28, 762–766.

Barnard, R., Edgerton, V., and Peter, J. Effects of exercise on skeletal muscle. II. Biochemical and histochemical properties. *Journal of Applied Physiology.* 1970, 28, 767–770.

Buchthal, F., and Schmalbruch, H. Contraction times and fiber types in intact human muscle. *Acta Physiologic Scandinavica.* 1970, 79, 435–452.

Clark, H. Cable tension strength tests. Springfield, Mass.: Brown and Murphy, 1953.

Hoffman, T. W., Stauffer, R. W., and Jackson, A. S. Sex differences in strength. *American Journal of Sport Medicine,* in Press.

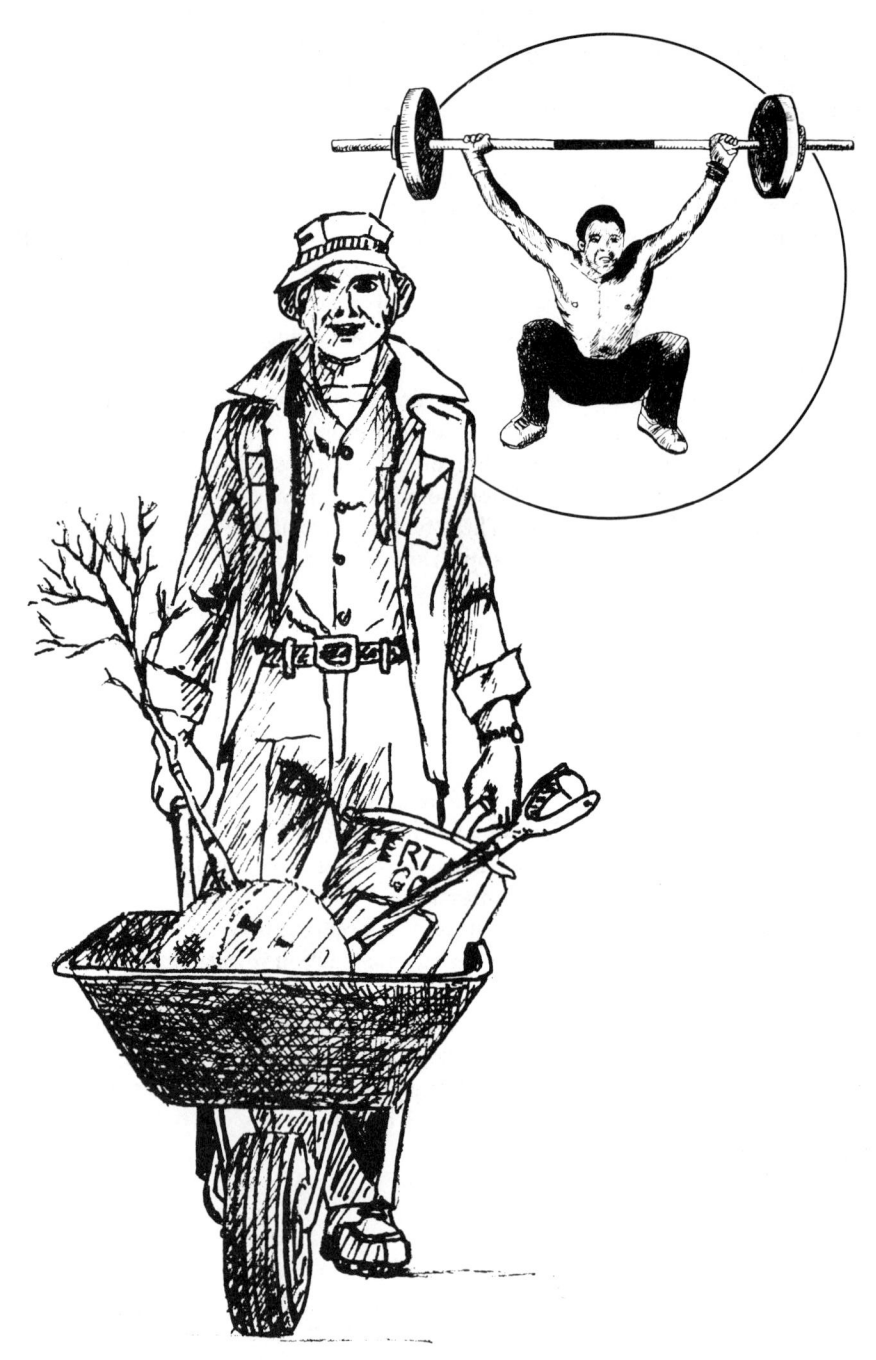

MUSCULAR STRENGTH

PERSONAL APPRAISAL No. 5
Muscular Strength

Physical activity requiring muscular contraction of greater intensity than the normal demands of daily living is essential to the development of muscular strength. This contributes to the development of an efficient, strong and durable body. Additionally, improved muscular tone will result in producing a more pleasing appearance and a sense of well-being.

Muscular strength is measured by computing the degree of force which the muscle can produce. Force is dependent upon the size and number of muscle fibers brought into action at any one time. Regular, progressive resistive activity has a profound positive effect on muscular strength. As a result of the overload principle, muscle and tendon fiber increase in diameter (hypertrophy), which permits the application of greater force and tension.

Unlike a machine which wears out with continued use, the human body thrives on activity. Disuse of the body has an adverse effect upon the muscular system. It can be noted that muscles of an arm or leg atrophy or deteriorate when placed in a cast. While this dramatic example demonstrates how atrophy occurs in a relatively short period of time, in effect this is what is happening throughout all muscles of the body when they are not used adequately.

This appraisal is designed to assist you in determining the levels of strength which are available in your major muscle groups. It will also hold major implications for a program of remediation.

Equipment and Facilities

    A. Hand Dynamometer

    B. Adjustable Barbells

    C. Multi-Stationed Progressive Resistance Machine

        1. Bench Press Station

        2. Leg Press Station

        3. Curl Station

        4. Latissimus Dorsi Station

        5. Military Press Station

        6. Hamstring Station

Procedures

    A. Follow the instructions provided for each test item. Have a clear understanding of the movement necessary for each item before the maximum effort is applied.

    B. Warm up with stretching and use minimal resistance while practicing each of the movements.

C. Before attempting each test item, estimate as accurately as possible the maximal resistance which can be succesfully lifted. After the first attempt, add or decrease the resistance appropriately in preparation for the second attempt.
D. Record the total amount of resistance successfully lifted in each of the following:

Test Item	Maximal Resistance Successfully Lifted
1. *Right Grip*—Set hand dynamometer gauge to "0" and place gauge facing palm. Perform maximal hand contraction. Do not touch body with hand during test.	
2. *Left Grip*—Test the left hand as in item No. 1.	
3. *Bench Press*—Lie in a supine position. Shoulder width grip—extend arms until elbows are locked and lower resistance to starting position.	
4. *Leg Press*—Extend legs until the knees lock and return resistance to starting position.	
5. *Curl*—Stand with palms forward, shoulder width grip, arms fully extended, elbows close to side. Flex lower arm, lifting bar to shoulder height and lower to starting position. Be sure to keep back straight throughout entire motion.	
6. *Latissimus Pull Down*—Assume kneeling position, with arms fully extended over head. While using a wide grip, pull the bar to back of neck and return to the starting position.	
7. *Military Press*—Stand with the resistance resting at shoulder level. While using a shoulder width grip, extend arms upward until the elbows are locked and lower to starting position.	
8. *Leg Curl*—Prone position, curl the lower leg until it breaks a vertical plane and lower to starting position.	

DEVIL'S BLOCK

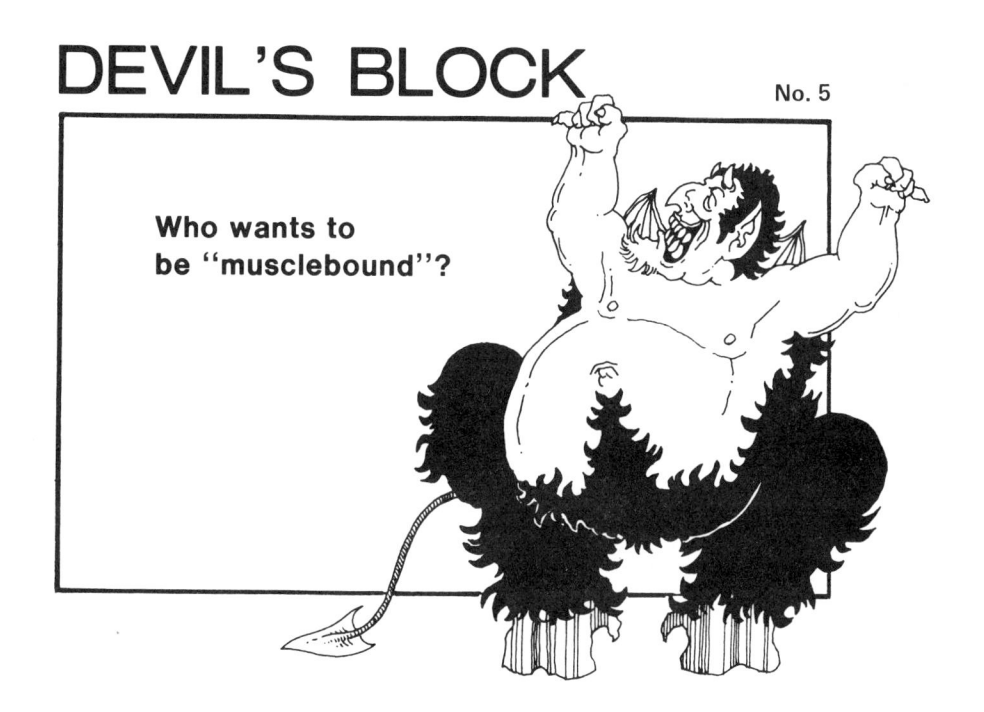

No. 5

Who wants to be "musclebound"?

EVALUATION REPORT
Personal Appraisal No. 5

Name _____

Date _____

Lifetime Participation

I. *Title:* Muscular Strength

II. *Objective*

III. *Results*

Circle Test Items Passed

Item No.	1	2	3	4	5	6	7	8	
Total Resistance									
Male	130	130	90% Body Wt.	180% Body Wt.	50% Body Wt.	60% Body Wt.	65% Body Wt.	45% Body Wt.	Minimal Resistance to Pass Test
Female	80	80	75%	150%	40%	50%	55%	40%	

Example:

Test item #3

Female:

   Body wt 120 lbs
       × .75
       90.00

To pass test—
   Bench press 90 lbs.

Scale

		Items Passed
1	Excellent Body Strength	8
2	Very Good	6-7
3	Good	4-5
4	Fair	3
5	Poor	2
6	Extremely Poor Strength	0-1

IV. *Analysis:*

1. Do the results of this appraisal substantiate or contradict your perceptions of your muscular strength held prior to taking this test? Explain!

2. Are you currently involved in activities that will maintain or increase your muscular strength?
    a. List activities.

3. Are you currently involved in activities that would be enhanced if your muscular strength were improved?
    a. List activities.

4. Describe your relative satisfaction or dissatisfaction with your present level of muscular strength.

V. *Implications:*

1. Do you intend to initiate a program designed to develop muscular strength? Describe the program.

2. Describe the manner in which increased muscular strength can be helpful in daily living.

6
MUSCULAR ENDURANCE

Muscular endurance can be defined as the ability of muscle tissue to persist in the repetition of submaximal contractions (isotonic) or sustained muscular contraction (isometric). This endurance can be accomplished either by the same motor units or by trading off of contractile responsibilities with other motor units. Endurance training seems to increase the oxidative or aerobic capacities of the individual fibers.

Two types of skeletal muscle fibers can be identified in human beings. The first, red (fast twitch) fibers, contract very quickly, however the contraction is of short duration. An individual with a high proportion of red fast twitch fibers has a great deal of potential speed and explosive power which are important attributes in sports such as track, basketball and football. The second type, white (slow twitch) fibers, are relatively slow in contracting. This fiber type is able to sustain contraction for longer periods of time. Individuals possessing high proportions of white fibers have potential in endurance activities such as distance running, soccer and swimming. Most of us have a balanced proportion of red and white fiber types and are by nature well suited for activities requiring both speed and endurance.

During rest and light exercise, the body utilizes fat as its primary source of energy for muscular contraction. Research indicates that endurance training will assist one in extracting greater percentages of energy from fat stores. During submaximal exercise, energy results from the oxidation of glycogen and fat. Stores of creatine phosphate, another energy source, and muscular glycogen are increased through training.

Muscular endurance and strength will increase through training, however, specific strength and endurance programs will produce specific results. This principle of *specificity of training* holds important implications for each of us. One must develop training programs designed to achieve specific results. For example a jogger who attempts to improve cardio-respiratory endurance and muscular endurance by following a program that will lead to running five miles in less than forty minutes will have fulfilled the training principle. Similarly a tennis player, recognizing the importance of endurance in the muscles of the forearm and hand, will train with many repetitions in the wrist curl and extension.

Muscular endurance plays an important role in successful participation in most sport activities. Its role in daily living is also important yet often overlooked by many. The ability of muscle groups to endure in contracting is important when one is involved in household chores such as carrying a full garbage can or shovelling snow. When a person's muscular endurance is insufficient for these types of tasks, muscle and joint strains and pulls may occur. In addition, as one tires or if undue fatigue results, the individual may change from positions insuring efficient body mechanics to faulty body positions which could result in serious joint injuries.

In the development of muscular endurance, physical activities which utilize the overload principle should be selected. Four categories of developmental exercise which increase muscular endurance valuable in sport activity include:

1. Resistance supplied by parts of the body, as in calisthenics.
2. Resistance supplied by inanimate objects, as in the use of free weights of multi-stationed resistance machines.
3. Resistance applied by body weight, as in chinning, use of peg boards, rope climbing.
4. Resistance applied by another individual as in wrestling, tug-of-war, acrobatics.

Selected References

Clarke, D. H., and Stull, G. A. Endurance training as a determinant of strength and fatigability. *Research Quarterly,* 1970, 41, 19–26.

Clarke, D. H. The influence on muscular fatigue patterns of the Intercontraction rest interval. *Medicine and Science in Sports.* 3:83–88, 1971.

Close, R. Dynamic properties of mammalian skeletal muscles. *Physiological Review,* 1972, 52, 129–197.

Holloszy, J. O. Adaption of skeletal muscle to endurance exercise. *Medicine and Science in Sports,* 1975, 7, 155–164.

Stull, G. A., and Clarke, D. H. High-resistance, low repetition training as a determiner of strength and fatigability. *Research Quarterly,* 1970, 41, 189–193.

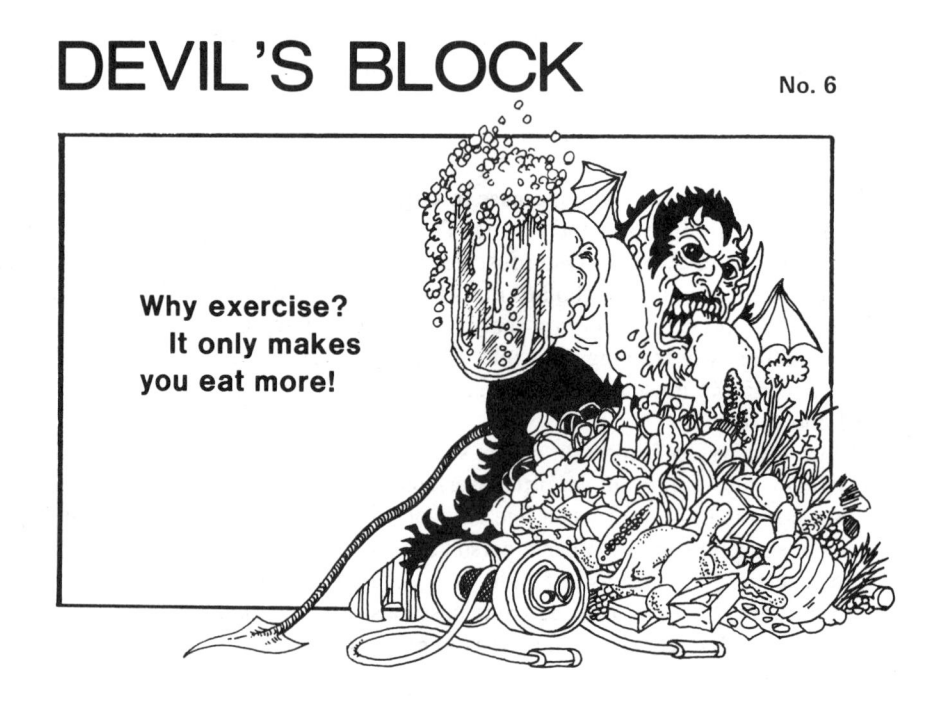

DEVIL'S BLOCK   No. 6

Why exercise? It only makes you eat more!

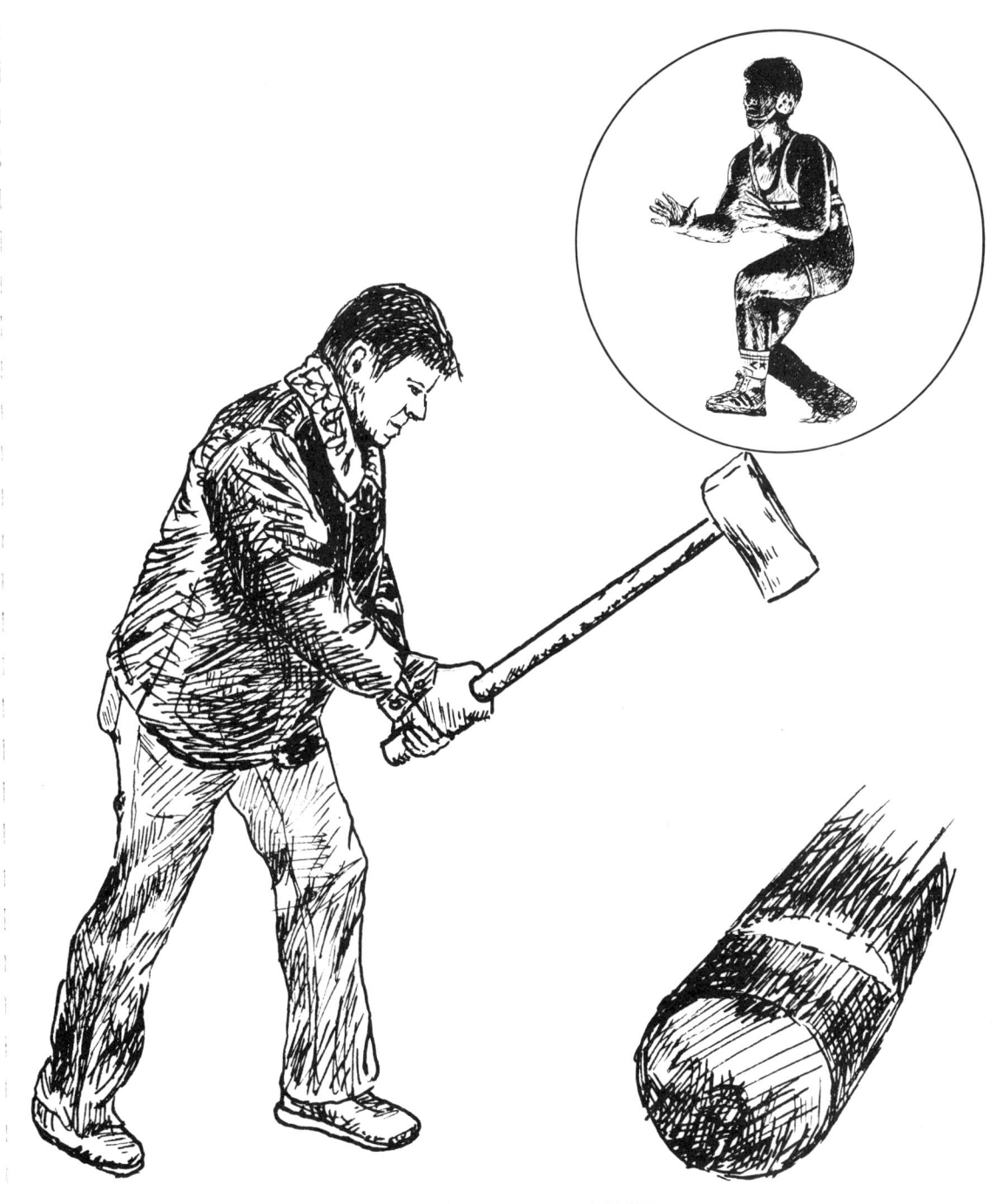

MUSCULAR ENDURANCE

PERSONAL APPRAISAL NO. 6
Muscular Endurance

During each day there are numerous occasions in which adequate amounts of muscular endurance will permit us to function more effectively. Safe and successful movement is often dependent upon our ability to delay and resist fatigue in the repetition or sustaining of muscular contraction. Our illustration on the opposite page shows a man sawing wood. How long can this chore be sustained before the muscles of the upper arm and shoulder tire to the point in which the effort must be terminated?

Do we have sufficient endurance to complete daily tasks calling for vigorous and repeated muscular contraction without resulting in undue fatigue or strain?

Since the fuel for muscular contraction is transported by the blood, there is an interrelationship between muscular endurance and the functioning of the cardio-respiratory system. Training produces an increased blood supply to the muscles. Additional capillaries are utilized and new capillary beds are created. This increased blood supply permits greater amounts of nutrients to be delivered to enlarged areas of muscle tissue. With continued muscular activity, and improved cardio-respiratory efficiency, the muscular system of the body is rendered more efficient and muscular endurance is increased.

Equipment and Facilities

   A. Adjustable Barbells

   B. Multi-Stationed Progressive Resistance Machine
   1. Bench Press Station
   2. Leg Press Station
   3. Curl Station
   4. Latissimus Pull Down Station
   5. Military Press Station
   6. Hamstring Station
   7. Chinning Station
   8. Dip Station

   C. Stopwatch

   D. Bench 18" High

   E. Masking Tape and Tape Measure

Procedures

A. Test I
   1. Stretch and perform light calisthenics which work the major muscle groups.
   2. Determine 75 percent of the maximum resistance lifted in each of the test items in Personal Appraisal 5, "Muscular Strength."
   3. Using the computed resistance, perform as many repetitions as possible in each of the test items, and record.

Test Item	Adjusted Resistance	Total Number of Repetitions
1. Bench Press		
2. Leg Press		
3. Curl		
4. Latissimus Pull Down		
5. Military Press		
6. Leg Curl		

B. Test II
1. Warm up—stretch and perform light calisthenics.
2. Perform and record the total number of repetitions for test items 1–5.
3. Record the number of seconds in which the body can remain sustained in a flexed hang position—test item 6.
4. Complete this appraisal while working with a partner.

Test Items	Total Number of Repetitions
1. *Chins*—Arms fully extended with palms forward—lift body until chin is above the bar—lower the body until arms are fully extended.	
2. *Dips*—Support body with arms fully extended at sides—lower body until shoulders are lower than elbows—lift body to starting position.	
3. *Sit-ups*—(1 Minute) Supine position—heels drawn to buttocks—knees apart—fingers interlocked behind neck—raise upper body until elbows touch midpoint of lower leg—lower body to starting position.	
4. *Push-ups*—Feet elevated on 18″ bench—front support position—arms shoulder width apart—fingers forward—lower body until chin touches floor—raise to starting position.	
5. *Vertical Jump*—Take maximum vertical jump and mark on wall—place a second mark 2″ lower—start vertical jumps in rhythm—1 jump every 3 seconds—count the number of jumps until the touch falls below the lower mark—execute each jump without approach step.	
6. *Flexed Hang* (No. of Seconds)—Hang from bar in flexed hang position. (Position—Arms flexed with chin above bar) Hold position until chin falls below hand level—record total number of seconds.	

EVALUATION REPORT
Personal Appraisal No. 6

Name _____

Date _____

Lifetime Participation

   I. *Title:* Muscular Endurance

  II. *Objective:*

 III. *Results:*

    A. Test I:

Circle Test Items Passed

Item No.	1	2	3	4	5	6
Total Number of Repetitions						
Minimal Reps to Pass Test	\multicolumn{6}{c}{Twelve Repetitions in Each Test Item}					

    B. Test II:

Circle Test Items Passed

	Item No.	1	2	3	4	5	6
	Total Number of Repetitions						sec.
Minimal Repetitions to Pass Test	Men	6	6	35	15	15	25 sec.
	Women	3	3	25	8	12	15 sec.

NOTE: If only one test is used—use column I. If both tests are completed, use column II.

Scale	I Test Items Passed	II Test Items Passed
1 Excellent Muscle Endurance	6	11–12
2 Very Good	5	9–10
3 Good	4	7–8
4 Fair	3	5–6
5 Poor	2	3–4
6 Extemely Poor Endurance	1	1–2

IV. *Analysis*

1. Has muscular endurance become significant as a result of completing this personal appraisal? Explain.

2. If you have completed test I and II, compare results.
    a. Are the results of each test similar? yes   no
       In what manner?

    b. Are the results of each test dissimilar? yes   no
       In what manner?

EVALUATION REPORT
Personal Appraisal No. 6

Name _____

Date _____

Lifetime Participation

  I. *Title:* Muscular Endurance

  II. *Objective:*

  III. *Results:*

    A. Test I:

Circle Test Items Passed

Item No.	1	2	3	4	5	6
Total Number of Repetitions						
Minimal Reps to Pass Test	Twelve Repetitions in Each Test Item					

    B. Test II:

Circle Test Items Passed

	Item No.	1	2	3	4	5	6
	Total Number of Repetitions						sec.
Minimal Repetitions to Pass Test	Men	6	6	35	15	15	25 sec.
	Women	3	3	25	8	12	15 sec.

NOTE: If only one test is used—use column I. If both tests are completed, use column II.

Scale	I Test Items Passed	II Test Items Passed
1 Excellent Muscle Endurance	6	11–12
2 Very Good	5	9–10
3 Good	4	7–8
4 Fair	3	5–6
5 Poor	2	3–4
6 Extemely Poor Endurance	1	1–2

IV. *Analysis*

1. Has muscular endurance become significant as a result of completing this personal appraisal? Explain.

2. If you have completed test I and II, compare results.
   a. Are the results of each test similar?   yes   no
      In what manner?

   b. Are the results of each test dissimilar?   yes   no
      In what manner?

Procedures

A. Test I
   1. Stretch and perform light calisthenics which work the major muscle groups.
   2. Determine 75 percent of the maximum resistance lifted in each of the test items in Personal Appraisal 5, "Muscular Strength."
   3. Using the computed resistance, perform as many repetitions as possible in each of the test items, and record.

Test Item	Adjusted Resistance	Total Number of Repetitions
1. Bench Press		
2. Leg Press		
3. Curl		
4. Latissimus Pull Down		
5. Military Press		
6. Leg Curl		

B. Test II
   1. Warm up—stretch and perform light calisthenics.
   2. Perform and record the total number of repetitions for test items 1–5.
   3. Record the number of seconds in which the body can remain sustained in a flexed hang position—test item 6.
   4. Complete this appraisal while working with a partner.

Test Items	Total Number of Repetitions
1. *Chins*—Arms fully extended with palms forward—lift body until chin is above the bar—lower the body until arms are fully extended.	
2. *Dips*—Support body with arms fully extended at sides—lower body until shoulders are lower than elbows—lift body to starting position.	
3. *Sit-ups*—(1 Minute) Supine position—heels drawn to buttocks—knees apart—fingers interlocked behind neck—raise upper body until elbows touch midpoint of lower leg—lower body to starting position.	
4. *Push-ups*—Feet elevated on 18″ bench—front support position—arms shoulder width apart—fingers forward—lower body until chin touches floor—raise to starting position.	
5. *Vertical Jump*—Take maximum vertical jump and mark on wall—place a second mark 2″ lower—start vertical jumps in rhythm—1 jump every 3 seconds—count the number of jumps until the touch falls below the lower mark—execute each jump without approach step.	
6. *Flexed Hang* (No. of Seconds)—Hang from bar in flexed hang position. (Position—Arms flexed with chin above bar) Hold position until chin falls below hand level—record total number of seconds.	

3. Are you currently involved in activities that will increase or maintain your levels of muscular endurance?

   a. List activities

4. Are you currently involved in activities that will be enhanced if you were to increase your muscular endurance?

   a. List activities

5. State your relative satisfaction or dissatisfaction with your present state of muscular endurance.

V. *Implications:*
   1. Do you feel it is important to increase your muscular endurance? Describe the program you intend to follow.

   2. How can increased levels of muscular endurance be helpful in your daily life.

SECONDARY COMPONENTS OF CONDITIONING

Chapter 7   Motor Performance Abilities
- Speed: Personal Appraisal No. 7
- Coordination: Personal Appraisal No. 8
- Agility: Personal Appraisal No. 9
- Balance: Personal Appraisal No. 10
- Explosive Power: Personal Appraisal No. 11

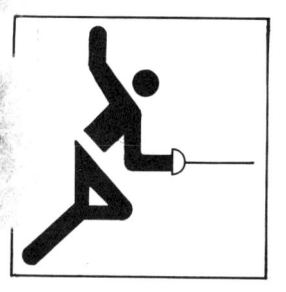

7
MOTOR PERFORMANCE ABILITIES

This area of conditioning consists of a number of abilities that influence the quality of performance of motor tasks. These abilities; speed, coordination, agility, balance, and explosive power function in permitting us to carry on efficient movement in our daily routines. To an extent heredity has predetermined the potential we possess in each of these areas. Each of these abilities can be developed through skill practice and training.

Each of us can benefit from the development of these abilities by being able to function more efficiently in the performance of the simple and complex tasks of daily living. Improved motor performance is critical to the athlete who seeks exceptional motor skills as well as the individual whose livelihood depends upon safe and efficient movement. As skills become refined, we tend to realize greater success in competitive as well as noncompetitive endeavors.

Those of us concerned with the physical and skill development of youth must realize the need for training and practice to reflect upon the improvement of speed, coordination, agility, balance and explosive power which are discussed below.

Speed

Speed, often referred to as *Movement Time,* is the interval of time in which the body or its extremities can move from one position to another. *Reaction Time* is an integral part of speed and can be defined as the interval of time necessary to initiate a response to a stimulus. Reaction time, then, is the time necessary for contraction of muscles at the start of a sprint in response to the starter's gun.

Ability to cover a prescribed distance in a certain amount of time is a result of two factors. The first is how fast you can accelerate from a standstill. This acceleration involves the first five or ten yards. Reaction and explosive power are important ingredients in this action. The second is the maximal movement rate, or the top speed that is finally generated. These two factors involved in speed are not necessarily related. An individual may be a proficient sprinter with a poor start because of excellent maximal movement rate. Conversely success may also be achieved in speed events with a quickness at the start and only an average maximal movement rate. As an example some individuals are proficient in football, tennis and badminton (utilizing quick starts) and yet do not perform well in the 100 yd. dash.

Factors that influence speed:

- Body mechanics: Body mechanics are important in speed. The proper arm action, leg action, angles of body as well as foot placement are critical in providing an efficiency of movement. Speed is generally increased through an improvement in body mechanics as excessive motion is reduced or virtually eliminated.
- Flexibility: Flexibility may play a role in improving speed by promoting more effective movement such as increasing the length of stride.
- Strength: Research has demonstrated that increases in strength are associated with significant gains in movement speed. Leg strength contributing additional drive is an example of this value.

For most of us, except those whose livelihoods or recreational pursuits demand speed and reaction time, the development of these two qualities is relatively unimportant. Athletes in most sport activities realize that speed and reaction time are extremely important as they strive towards excellence.

Coordination

Coordination is the common denominator of all motor ability components. Coordination involves the nervous skeletal and muscle systems, and the senses of sight, feeling and hearing. Kinesthenic sense, which is the awareness of the position and balance of the body is an additional consideration. Coordination then is the relationship of the motor abilities working together to make movement efficient, whether it involves typing, running, participating in sports, writing, driving a car, walking, etc.

Minimal levels of coordination are necessary in our daily lives. Through practice the specific examples of coordination such as shooting a pistol, hitting a nail on the head, writing or typing can be improved.

Balance

Balance is a complex aspect of coordination involving reflexes, vision, the inner ear, skeletal-muscular system and the cerebellum. Balance is an integral factor in kinesthetic sense. There are three types of balance: stationary; dynamic; and balancing of objects.

- Stationary balance: Involves the maintenance of equilibrium in a fixed position. An example would be a person standing on a ladder or performing a hand balance.
- Dynamic balance: Is the ability to maintain equilibrium during movement. Examples would include walking on a scaffold while painting and executing a cartwheel in tumbling.
- Object Balance: Infers the ability to balance objects with segments of the body. Balancing a yardstick on the end of a finger or a ball on the back of the hand are examples of object balancing.

Each of these forms of balance can be improved through the practice of skills that require their specific use. We take balance for granted yet it provides us with the ability to remain erect, walk without falling and hold or lift objects. Those handicapped with a disorder resulting in a loss of balance have a great deal of difficulty with everyday tasks.

Agility

Agility can be defined as the ability to change direction quickly and efficiently and generally requires nimbleness of movement. This particular component of motor ability is very important in most sport activities which are dependent upon quick changes of gross movements, i.e. ballet and basketball. Because of this, agility is an important factor in successful motor performance. A reasonable degree of agility is also desirable for daily activities such as walking across a busy street. For the most part the average individual does not need to develop agility to a great extent, although agility may prove vital in emergency situations which call for quick movements and change of direction.

Like balance and coordination, agility will improve through practice of specific movements which involve changes in direction.

Explosive Power

Explosive power is directly related to strength, one of the primary components of conditioning. We can think of explosive power as the ability to produce maximum muscular force in the shortest period of time. Concisely explosive power is a combination of speed and strength in which the ability to apply strength in a sudden movement is paramount. We can express explosive power with a formula.

$$\text{POWER} = \frac{\text{Force} \times \text{Distancce}}{\text{Time}}$$

To illustrate this concept, we can observe two persons bench press 200 pounds, a distance of 30 inches. One person completes the press in 5 seconds, while the other completes the press in 2 1/2 seconds. The latter has demonstrated twice the power of the former subject.

Pushing a car stuck in sand and starting to move a loaded wheelbarrow are examples of home activities utilizing explosive power.

This motor ability is an extremely important factor in the succcessful performance of many sports. It can be developed by promoting the muscular strength involved in a specific movement and increasing the speed of skill execution. As examples:

A basketball player can increase jumping ability (explosive power) by rapidly performing a series of vertical jumps while wearing a weighted vest. Each jump should be executed as rapidly as possible without sacrificing technique and full range of movement.

The shot putter interested in improving explosive power would train with maximum resistance and minimal repetitions (1–5), and run sprints emphasizing quick starts. This combination is designed to increase strength and speed.

Selected References

Dillman, C. J. Effect of leg segmental movements on foot velocity during the recovery phase of running. R. C. Nelson and C. A. Morehouse (Eds.) Biomechanics IV. Baltimore: University Park Press, 1974.

Halverson, L. E., Roberton, M. A., and Harper, C. J. Current research in motor development. *Journal of Research and Development in Education,* 1973, 6, 56–70.

Henery, F. M. and Trafton, I. R. The velocity curve of sprint running. *Research Quarterly,* 1951, 22, 404–422.

Kaneko, M. The relationship between force, velocity and mechanical power in human muscle. *Research Journal of Physical Education* (Japan), 1970, 14, 141–145.

Whiting, H. T. A. Acquiring Ball Skill: A psychological interpretation. Philadelphia: Lea and Febiger, 1969.

DEVIL'S BLOCK No. 7

Modern inventions have made the necessity of physical fitness obsolete. Besides we live by our intellect!

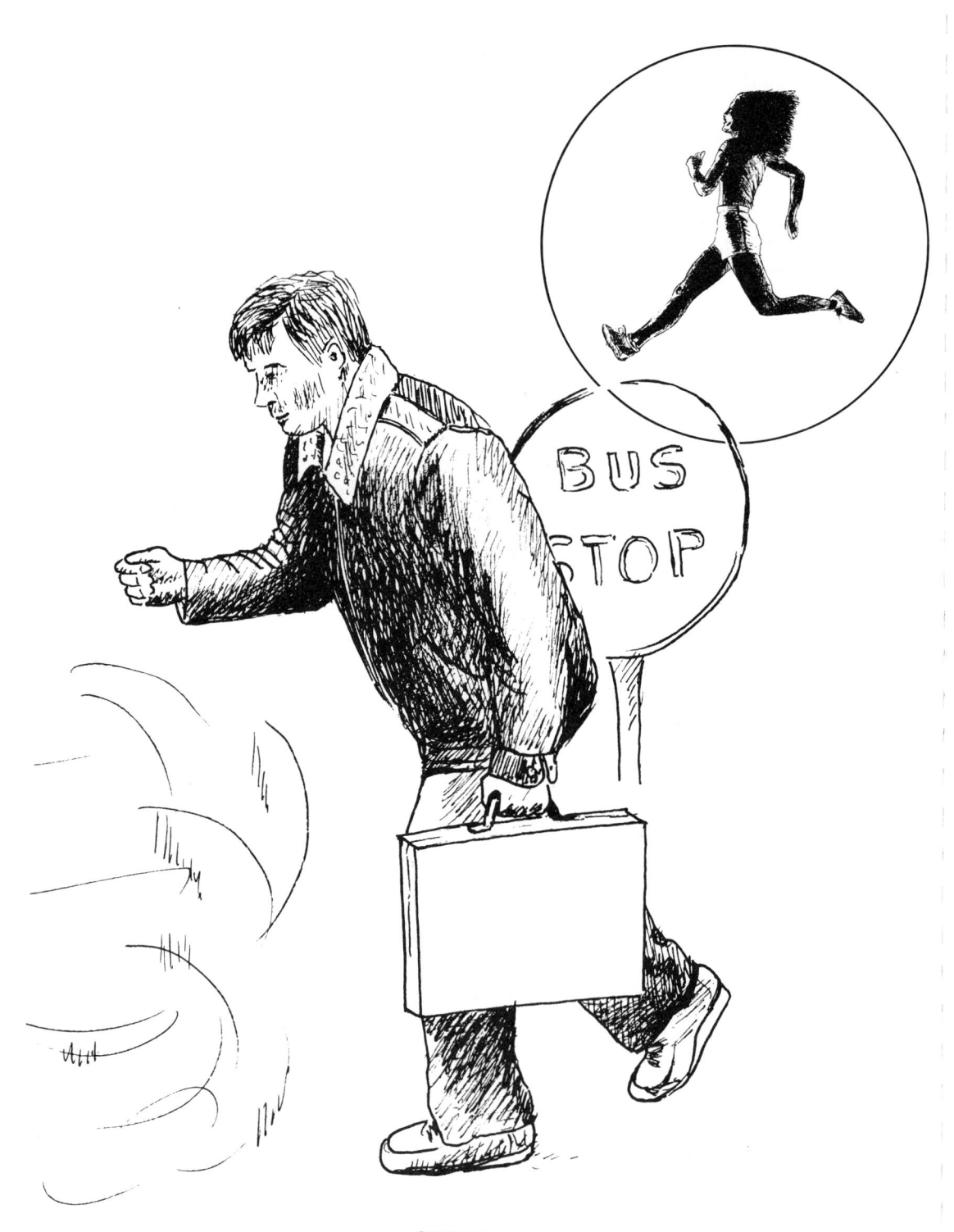

SPEED

PERSONAL APPRAISAL NO. 7
Speed

Speed is usually evaluated in terms of distance, however, it is possible to determine one's top speed in miles per hour and one's rate of acceleration in reaching maximum speed. This is an uncommon procedure. Speed is commonly computed by measuring the elapsed time it takes an individual to travel a specific distance. This occurs in track, bobsledding, speed skating, swimming and a host of other activities. Occasionally speed is computed as the average of time over distance as in a 180 mile-per-hour average at the Indianapolis Speedway.

One may be able to produce fast speeds in short distances yet move slowly in longer distances. For our purposes, we will measure speed in terms of the sprint or short distance. Speed and reaction time are important factors in most sports.

Equipment and Facilities
   A. Stopwatch

   B. Preferably a macadum surface marked at 40 yards with enough deceleration space for safety

Procedures
1. Run the forty-yard dash as fast as you can for a time
2. Start whenever you feel ready
3. Timer will start the stopwatch as soon as the runner initiates movement

_____Time

EVALUATION REPORT
Personal Appraisal No. 7

Name _____

Date _____

Lifetime Participation

I. *Laboratory Title:* Speed

II. *Objective:*

III. *Results:*

40-yard dash time _____

Compare your time with others in terms of the standards below:

	Men	Scale	Women
1	4.5–4.8	Excellent	5.0–5.2
2	4.9–5.0	Good	5.3–5.4
3	5.1–5.2	Above average	5.5–5.6
4	5.3–5.4	Average	5.7–5.9
5	5.5–5.7	Below average	6.0–6.2
6	5.8–6.0	Poor	6.3–6.5

IV. *Analysis:*

    1. In your opinion are the results of this personal appraisal significant? Explain.

    2. Describe the experiences you have had in which increased speed could have been to your advantage.

    3. Does your body size and shape exert a positive or negative influence over your ability to move quickly? Explain!

    4. State your relative satisfaction or dissatisfaction with your ability to move quickly.

V. *Implications:*
   1. Describe activities that you are interested in which would improve your speed.

   2. Describe ways in which speed can be an important factor in your life.

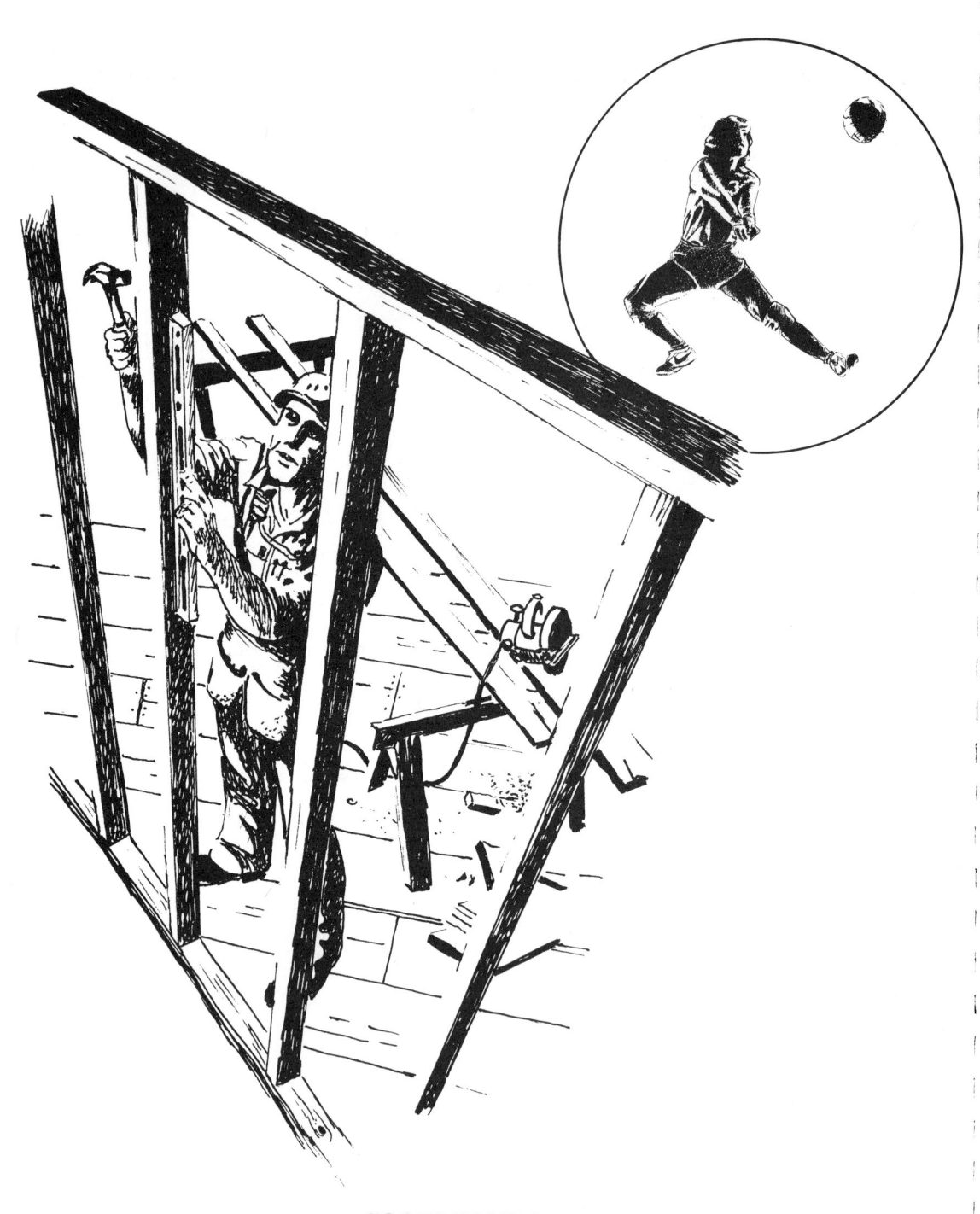

COORDINATION

PERSONAL APPRAISAL NO. 8
Coordination

Coordination is a motor performance quality that we often take for granted, however it is the basis for all efficient and meaningful movement. Coordination occurs in segments as in the precision of a musician's fingers when playing a Bach Fugue, or the deftness of a surgeon while performing a delicate operation. It also occurs in unified and controlled total body movement experienced by the breast stroke swimmer, and the eye, arm and leg motion of the punt in football. Evaluation of coordination of body segments and total body movement is an extremely difficult task. Our tests are designed to show specific eye-hand and eye-foot coordination. However, they may also suggest implications regarding the efficiency of total body movement.

Equipment and Facilities

   A. 8" Rubber Playground Balls (suggested)

   B. Two Tennis Balls

   C. Softball

Procedures

Check if test is successfully completed

   A. Practice each item once before taking test

   B. Two Foot Pick-up

     1. Place an 8" playground ball between feet. While placing pressure against the ball with the inside ankles, jump into the air thrusting the ball upward and catch with the hands.   1. _____

   C. One Foot Pick-up

     1. Place the toe of the right foot on the top of an 8" playground ball and extend the foot downward creating back spin on the ball. As the ball rolls up on the toe, lift the foot thrusting the ball upward and catching it in the right hand. Perform this test with the left foot.   2. _____
                                                                                                                         3. _____

   D. Simple Juggle

     1. While holding a softball in one hand and a tennis ball in the other, throw both balls simultaneously up into the air a minimum of one foot and catch in the opposite hand. This should be repeated five times in a rhythmical manner.   4. _____

E. Wall Bounce

   1. Hold a tennis ball in each hand and stand approximately one yard from a wall. Using an underhand motion, throw both balls against the wall and catch them on the rebound. This should be repeated five times in a rhythmical manner.

Check if test is successfully completed
_____

5. _____

EVALUATION REPORT
Personal Appraisal No. 8

Name _____

Date _____

Lifetime Participation

I. *Title:* Coordination

II. *Objective:*

III. *Results:*

Circle Test Items Passed

1 2 3 4 5

Score
5—Excellent
4—Above Average
3—Average
2—Below Average
0–1—Poor

IV. *Analysis:*

1. Provide the reasons for failing specific test items.

2. Relate any experiences you have had in which increased coordination would have been to your advantage.

V. *Implications:*

1. Describe any endeavors that you currently engage in that would be enhanced if your coordination were improved.

2. Are there any activities you would enjoy participating in, which would result in improved coordination.

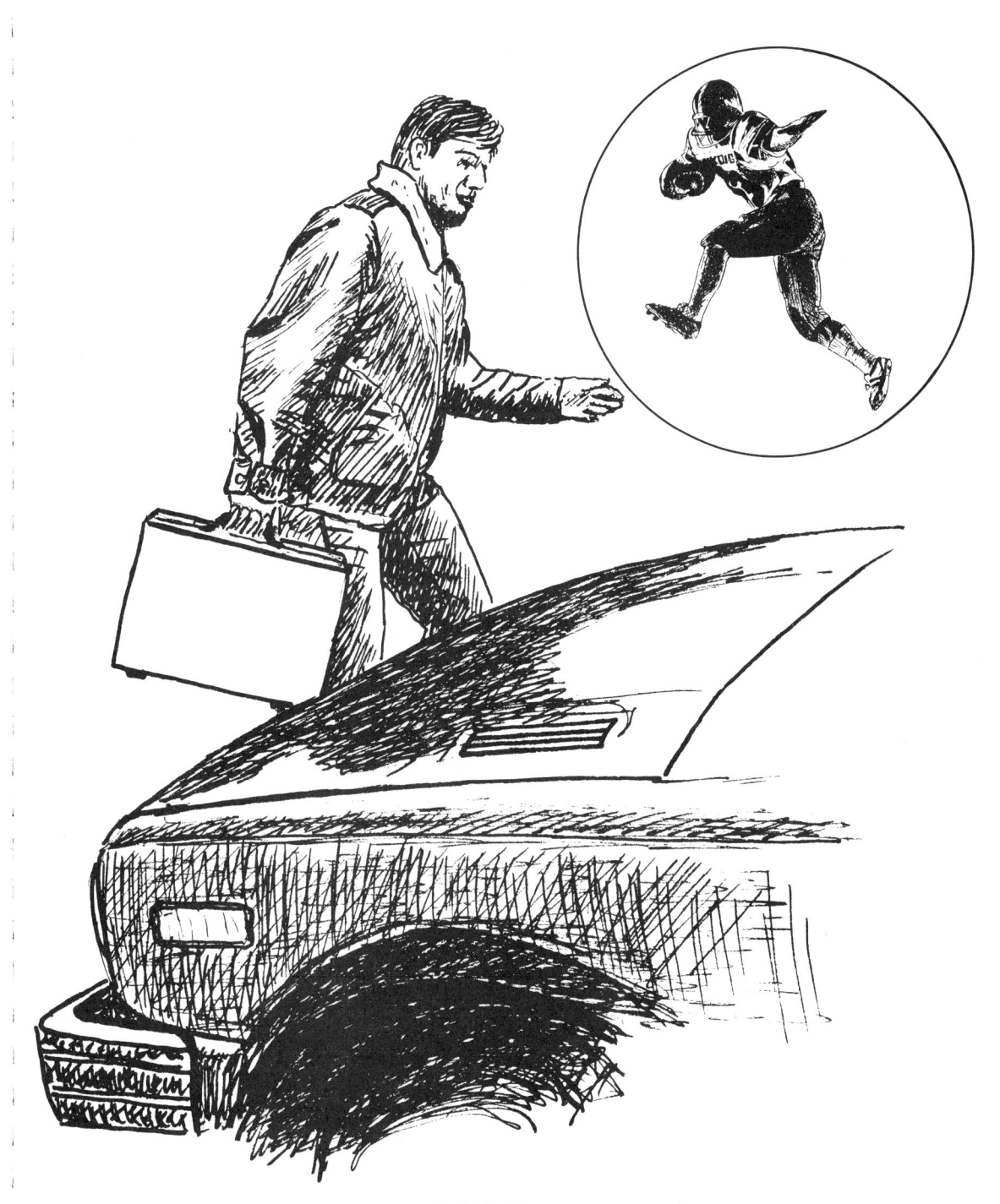

AGILITY

PERSONAL APPRAISAL NO. 9
Agility

Agility is a motor performance ability that is concerned with quick and efficient change of direction. Aspects of balance and coordination can be found in virtually all body movements requiring agility. Although high levels of agility may not be required for successful daily living, it is an important factor in many athletic activities. Adequate levels of agility can be measured by completing the following tests.

Equipment and Facilities
   A. Stopwatch
   B. Running Area—minimum 10′ × 20′
   C. Marking Tape

Procedures
   A. Test A (Shuttle Run)
      1. With tape, mark off three 6′ parallel lines 7 1/2′ apart.
      2. During shuttle run, change of direction is initiated by touching the line or area beyond mid-line with the hand.
      3. Start by straddling the middle line. When ready follow diagram and directions:
         a. *Diagram*

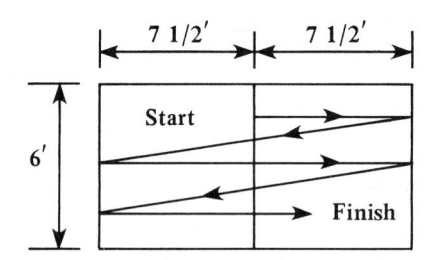

         b. *Directions*
            (1) Sprint to right line and touch
            (2) Change direction to far left line and touch
            (3) Change direction and sprint to far right line and touch.
            (4) Change direction and sprint to far left line and touch.
            (5) Change direction and finish by sprinting across mid line.

4. Timer will start stopwatch on initial movement. Make sure each line or surface beyond line is touched with the hands and record time after the final 7 1/2′ dash. Upon completion of the test, you will have run three 15′ dashes and two 7 1/2′ dashes.

_____ Time

B. Test B (Jack Springs)

1. Jump up from floor with legs apart in a "v" position—touch hands to toes at waist level keeping legs straight. Repeat five times in succession.

_____ (Yes-No)

EVALUATION REPORT
Personal Appraisal No. 9

Name _____

Date _____

Lifetime Participation

  I. *Laboratory Title:* Agility

 II. *Objective:*

III. *Results:*

    A. Shuttle Run Time _____

    B. 5 consecutive Jack Springs (Yes-No) _____

Shuttle Run Equivalencies

	Men		Women
1	−5.0	Excellent	5.1–5.8
2	5.1–5.8	Above average	5.9–6.4
3	5.9–6.4	Average	6.5–6.8
4	6.5–6.8	Below average	6.9–7.3
5	6.9–	Poor	7.4–

IV. *Analysis:*

    1. Can you find significance in the results of this personal appraisal? Explain.

    2. Compare the results of test item A and test item B. Explain any differences.

    3. Describe the experiences you have had in which increased agility would have been to your advantage.

V. *Implications:*

    1. Describe any endeavors that you currently engage in which would be enchanced if your agility were improved.

    2. Describe the activities that you would be interested in which would result in improved agility.

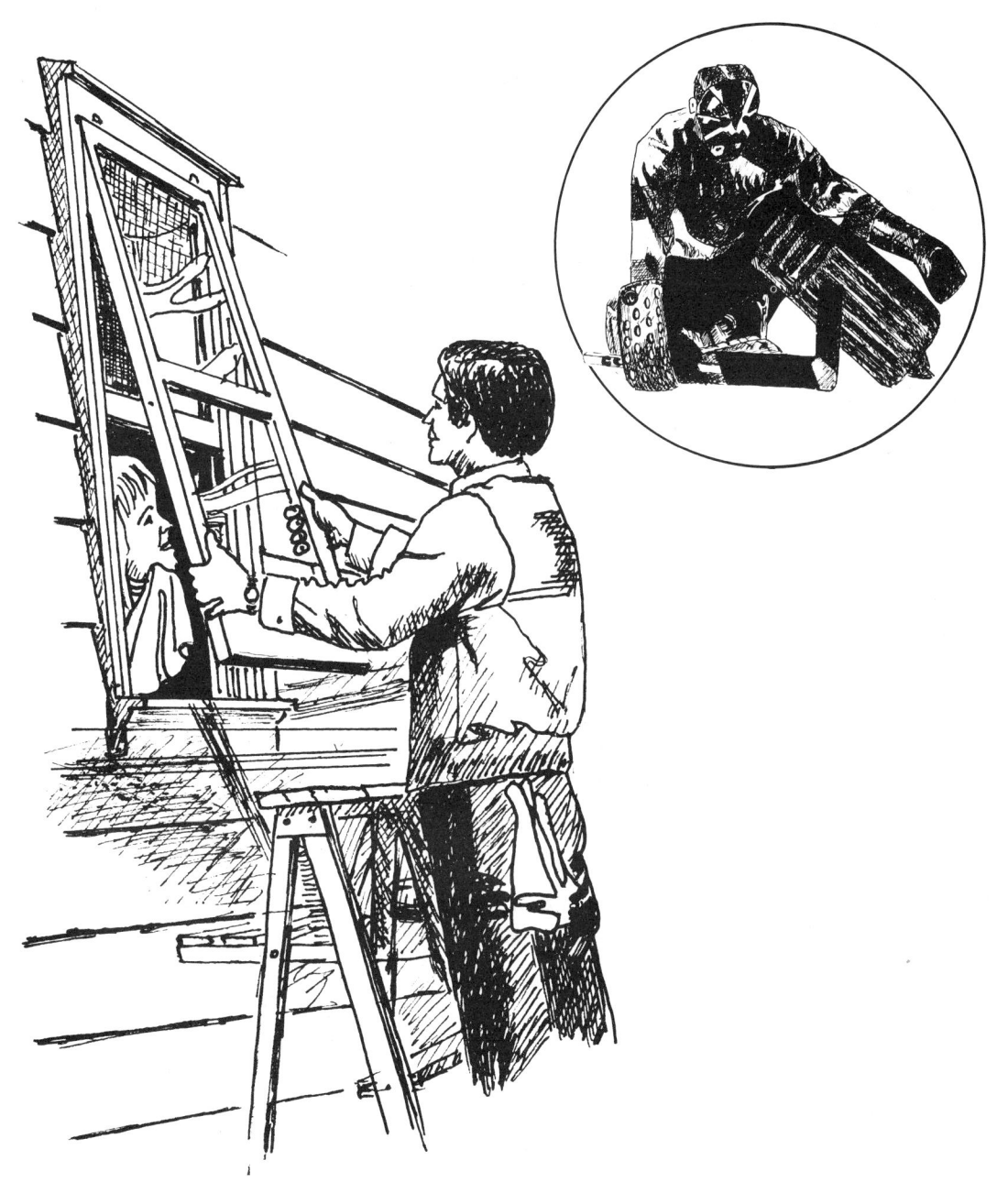

BALANCE

PERSONAL APPRAISAL NO. 10
Balance

We often consider balance as an ability necessary only for the circus performer, gymnast and high steel construction worker. Of course, these individuals require exceptional ability in maintaining equilibrium. All of us, however, utilize this basic ingredient which allows us to assume efficient stationary and dynamic body positions with smoothness and grace.

Stationary balance implies the maintenance of equilibrium while in a fixed position. Dynamic balance indicates the maintenance of equilibrium during total body locomotion. An additional aspect of equilibrium, not previously mentioned, is that of balancing an object with segments of the body. Many examples of this ability are needed in household chores as well as athletics.

This personal appraisal will assist in evaluating whether or not you have adequate levels of balance in each of the categories mentioned above.

Equipment and Facilities

A. Stopwatch

B. 1" Width Tape at least seven yards in length

C. 3' Long 1/2" diameter pole (suggested)

D. 6" Playground ball.

Procedures

1. Work with partner during each test item.

2. Practice each item once before taking the test.

A. Test I—Sleeping Diver

1. Stand with feet shoulder width apart, arms extended in diver's approach position and eyes closed. Raise body by extending toes. Attempt to maintain balance in this position for as long as possible.

2. Partner—record the length of time the subject is able to maintain balance.

_____ sec.

B. Test II—Cross Over

1. Place 1" width tape on floor, stretching at least seven yards in length.

2. Perform entire test while standing on the balls of the feet.

3. Stand with the balls of the feet covering tape at the right end.

4. Take ten successive steps along tape by passing right foot over left and left behind right, etc.

5. Repeat the test by starting from the left end of the tape and reversing the stepping action of No. 4 above.
6. In order to pass, the toes must remain extended throughout with the balls of the feet as the only point of contact with the tape.
7. Note: Shoulders and hips should be parallel with the direction of the tape.

C. Test III—Object Balance
   1. With palm down, balance pole on back of left hand.
   2. Balance 6″ ball on instep of right foot, while standing on your left leg.
   3. Partner—record the length of time the subject was able to maintain each balance.

   1. _____ sec.

   2. _____ sec.

D. Test IV—Tipup (Squat Balance)
   1. Squat position. Place hands on floor, shoulder width apart, position legs so that inside of thighs rest against the elbows. Lean forward, keeping head up, until the feet clear the floor. The hands become the sole means of support.
   2. Partner—record the length of time the subject is able to maintain balance.

   _____ sec.

EVALUATION REPORT
Personal Appraisal No. 10

Name _____

Date _____

Lifetime Participation

I. *Title:* Balance

II. *Objective:*

III. *Results:*

	Pass	Fail	Items
A. Test I—sleeping driver			
Balance time	_____	_____	1
Passing time—20 sec.			
B. Test II—cross over			
Right to left	_____	_____	2
Left to right	_____	_____	3
C. Test III—object balance			
Left hand (20 sec.)	_____	_____	4
Right foot (10 sec.)	_____	_____	5
D. Test IV—tipup			
Passing time—8 sec	_____	_____	6

Scale

5-6—Excellent
4—Above Average
3—Average
2—Below Average
0-1—Poor

IV. *Analysis:*

    1. In what way is the completion of this personal appraisal meaningful to you? Explain.

    2. Provide reasons for any differences in the results of the test items.

V. *Implications:*

    1. Can you think of the ways in which improvement in balance would be to your advantage.

    2. Describe the types of activities that you would be interested in which would result in improved balance.

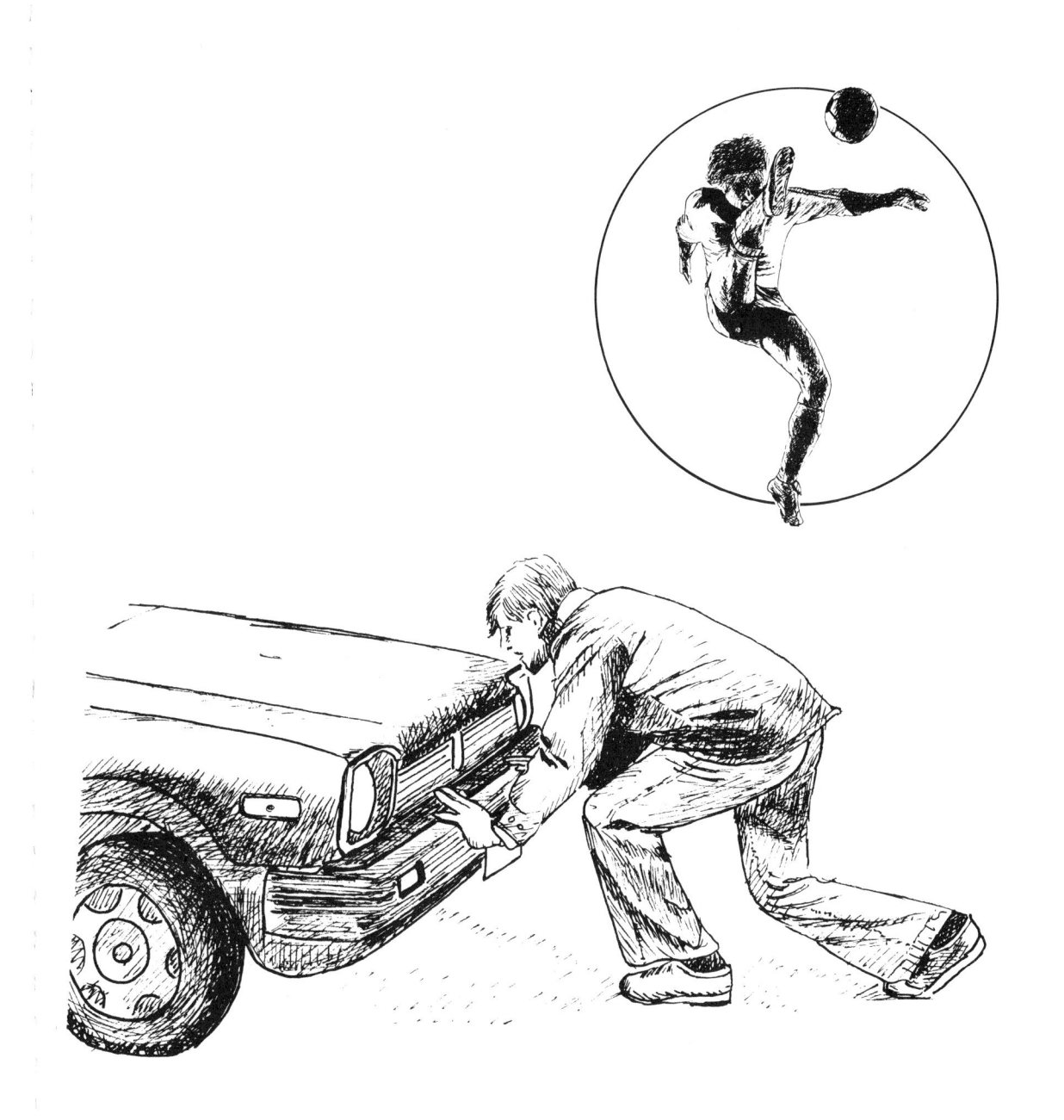

EXPLOSIVE POWER

PERSONAL APPRAISAL NO. 11
Explosive Power

Those endowed with high levels of explosive power have a decided advantage in performing physical skills. To be able to propel the body upward or outward from a stationary position with force and speed often provides the athlete with the winning edge. Individuals rise above the ordinary when they are able to unleash high levels of explosive power. The football lineman who uncoils and strikes before his opponent can react; the high-jumper who at the moment of truth literally seems to explode his body from the horizontal to the vertical plane; the sprinter who seems to be shot from a cannon as he releases himself from the starting block, are all examples of this quality.

Many believe explosive power is inherent in the individual. While it is true that high potential in this area may be due to hereditary or early environmental factors, each of us can increase explosive power through participation in a program of activity specifically designed for this purpose.

Equipment and Facilities
- A. Tape Measure
- B. Masking Tape
- C. Wall with no obstructions
- D. Tumbling Mat
- E. 15 lb.—medicine ball

Procedures
- A. Vertical Jump:
    1. Secure masking tape against wall—starting at 6′ in height and extending upward to 12′.
    2. The vertical jump is the differential between the subject's normal reach and the point touched after jumping upward.
    3. Stand at right angle to wall, touch side of body to wall, feet together, heels on floor, reach up with arm as high as possible—touch masking tape and mark.
    4. From this starting position, jump as high as you can and place mark at the highest point touched.
    5. Measure the distance between these two marks and record.
    6. Distance between first and second mark = _____ inches

B. Standing Long Jump:
   1. Mark a line on tumbling mat for the point of take off.
   2. Place both feet together—toes just touching the take off point.
   3. Jump as far as you can.
   4. At the completion of the jump, mark the point of body contact closest to the take off line (usually back of heel).
   5. Measure and record the distance from the take off line to the closest point of contact.

   _____Ft. _____Inches

C. Medicine Ball Thrust
   1. Sit with legs crossed—as close to starting line as possible.
   2. Hold medicine ball with two hands, in front of chest.
   3. Utilizing chest pass technique—pass the ball as far forward as possible.
   4. Mark point where the center of medicine ball touches the floor. Measure the distance ball is passed, from the starting line.
   5. After two attempts, record the greatest distance.

   _____Ft. _____Inches

EVALUATION REPORT
Personal Appraisal No. 11

Name _____

Date _____

Lifetime Participation

I. *Title:* Explosive Power

II. *Objective:*

III. *Results:*

    A. Verticle Jump   B. Standing Long Jump   C. Medicine Ball Thrust

    _____ inches   _____ ft _____ inches   _____ ft _____ inches

Vertical Jump Men	Vertical Jump Women	Scale		Horizontal Jump Men	Horizontal Jump Women
25" & above	21" & above	1	Outstanding	Height + 1'	Ht. + 9"
21"–24"	17"–20"	2	Excellent	Height + 9"	Ht. + 6"
17"–20"	13"–16"	3	Very good	Height + 6"	Ht. + 3"
13"–16"	9"–12"	4	Good	Height + 3"	Height
9"–12"	5"–8"	5	Fair	Height + 0"	Ht.–3"
5"–8"	–4"	6	Poor	Less than height	Less than ht.–3"

Medicine Ball Thrust			
Men		**Scale**	**Women**
12'6" +	1.	Outstanding	8'6" +
12' – 12'5"	2.	Excellent	8' – 8'5"
11'6" – 11'11"	3.	Very good	7'6" – 7'11"
11' – 11'5"	4.	Good	7' – 7'5"
10'6" – 10'11"	5.	Fair	6'6" – 6'11"
– 10'5"	6.	Poor	– 6'5"

IV. *Analysis:*

1. Are the results of this personal appraisal significant? Did any difference in explosive power occur between the upper and lower extremities? Explain.

2. If you scored in the excellent or outstanding range, describe the reasons which contributed to your success. If you scored average to poor, provide a rationale for your performance?

3. Describe any experiences you have had in which increased explosive power would have been to your advantage.

V. *Implications:*

1. Analyze the endeavors you presently engage in which would be enhanced if your explosive power were increased.

2. If improvement in explosive power becomes your objective, describe a program you would follow to improve this ability.

MAJOR INFLUENCES ON CONDITIONING

Chapter 8   Posture and Body Mechanics
                Personal Appraisal No. 12

Chapter 9   Weight Control
                Personal Appraisal No. 13

Chapter 10   Emotional Adjustment

Chapter 11   Chemical Influences

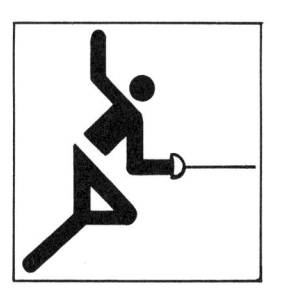

8
POSTURE AND BODY MECHANICS

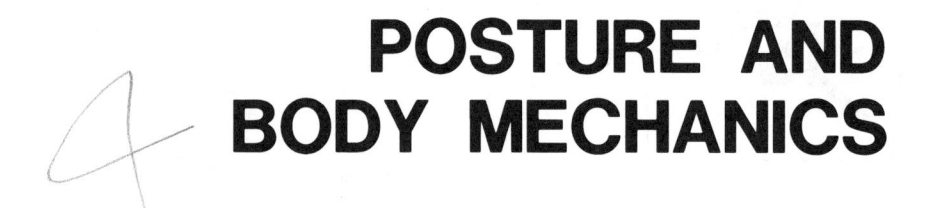

Would you be interested if someone should say to you, "At this moment, I have the immediate power to improve your appearance and the cost will be minimal?"

The truth is that each of us has this ability. One of the most efficient and economical ways to improve appearance is to concentrate on improving posture. Posture includes all of the body positions assumed during movement or while stationary. Posture is dynamic as well as static. It is a measure of the degree of efficiency of body movement and position. Total body efficiency is based upon the coordination of the nervous, skeletal, muscular and visceral systems. It is a function of the alignment of body segments and the distribution of weight over supporting structures. Because of individual differences, there is no single correct posture; however, certain principles are applicable to all.

As you are reading this, begin the following reactions: hold the head up high as the chin is drawn in, shoulders back as the chest is lifted, firm the abdomen. If you are sitting, push the hips toward the rear of the chair. Your personal appearance is now improved, and most importantly, you have assumed a more efficient body position. The problem now is to be able to maintain this body alignment for extended periods of time. To accomplish this, a degree of muscular strength, endurance, and tone is needed.

Throughout life, efficient movement is dependent to a great extent upon functional body structure. Posture and body mechanics play an important role in influencing performance potential. Standing, sitting and moving (dynamic posture), may be thought of as the alignment of body parts and segments. When correct posture is assumed, we help maintain the structural positioning for which the body was designed. Through continuous use of improper or negative alignment of body segments, a structural change or deviation may result. Apart from being unattractive, this deviation may result in limitations in normal ranges of movement, and even more importantly, dangerous pressure upon body organs. In addition, improper posture and body mechanics may result in strain, muscle pull, rupture, etc.

Body mechanics indicates the technique and body positioning used in performing motor tasks. When acceptable mechanics of movement are incorporated, we function more efficiently and are able to perform increased work for longer periods of time with less risk of injury. If we utilize faulty body mechanics while performing work, we tire more easily, become less efficient, and find ourselves more susceptible to injury.

The maintenance of correct posture is, to some extent, affected by the degree of muscular strength and endurance we possess. The human bi-ped position places a great demand on these qualities since we are constantly resisting the forces of gravity. Can you recall how easy it is to slip into poor sitting posture when you are tired? When muscles become fatigued, we tend to become careless and collapse into a position offering least resistance. With adequate muscular strength and endurance, assuming correct posture can be a simple and comfortable task.

Correct posture communicates a favorable impression to others. It indicates that one is conscientious regarding proper body alighment and structure. Research has indicated that posture reflects personality, self-esteem, and a degree of aggressiveness. Although the validity of this hypothesis may be questioned, from an esthetic viewpoint, correct posture is highly desirable.

The significance of proper body alignment becomes apparent in the following example: When the question is asked, *"What is middle age?"* The usual response to this question is to indicate chronological age (at age 30, 40, or 50). The age selected is usually in light of the age of the person responding to the question. To the nine year old, fifteen years of age is ancient. To the twenty-one year old, thirty-five years would be classified as "middle age."

In reality, "middle age" is that time in life when someone approaches you and tells you to stand up straight, hold your head up high, chin in, chest out, abdomen in—and your reply is, *"I already have."* If you respond in this fashion, you are now in a state of "physical middle age." The midsection of our body is extremely vital in countering the forces of gravity. When we lose abdominal muscle tone, we lose valuable structural support which helps the internal organs maintain functional position. Due to the lack of muscular control in failing to combat the forces of gravity, congestion of the internal viscera occurs. This problem results in physical ailments which are often attributed to middle age. This condition is not related to chronological age and may be experienced during early years. However, some adults avoid this degenerative process throughout life.

Postural Recommendations

If we incorporate logic and knowledge, assuming correct posture can be a relatively simple task. Muscular tone and strength assist us in maintaining good posture. Exercise programs designed to improve these qualities can be valuable if balanced muscular development results. Faulty alignment can occur from the stimulation of agonist muscle groups, while antagonist muscles are disregarded. Assuming correct posture in itself may be a form of exercise with a resultant increase in tone. Using appropriate techniques of body mechanics has a favorable effect on posture. Conversely, poor body mechanics, such as not bending at the knees when lifting objects from the floor, may result in strain, joint injury and postural deviations.

The following seven conditions will assist us in achieving and maintaining proper structural alignment of the body:

1. *High Head*—has the following chain reaction of increasing height, raising eyes off the ground, lifting chest, flattening the abdomen and straightening the back.
2. *Elevated Chest*—the chest cavity providing an enlarged area for the vital organs—i.e., lungs, heart, and stomach.
3. *Retracted Shoulders*—transfers the weight of the shoulder girdle off the chest, relieving pressure on the vital organs.
4. *Firm Abdomen*—provides support and proper placement of the internal viscera, resulting in efficient function.
5. *Flat Back*—a term used to describe a method aiding in the reduction of exaggerated spinal curves.

6. *Upward Pelvic Tilt*—It is a natural tendency for the pelvis to tilt forward and downward—this causes the abdominal organs to move forward—Sacro-Lumbar joints are strained and the body in general is forced out of proper alignment. To avoid this condition, there must be adequate muscular tone in the abdominal and gluteal regions.
7. *Feet Pointed Straight Forward*—mechanically this is the most efficient position for walking and running.

The following illustrations and brief descriptions emphasize the salient features of healthful posture:

Standing Posture (Front View) (A)

1. Straight head position
2. Parallel shoulders
3. Even hips
4. Feet pointed slightly out

Standing Posture (Back View) (C)

1. Straight head position
2. Head position aligned with vertebral column
3. Shoulders parallel
4. Even hips

Standing Posture (Side View) (B)

1. Aligment of the ear, shoulders, hips, knees, ankles

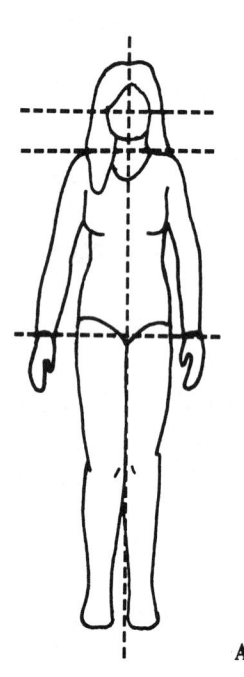

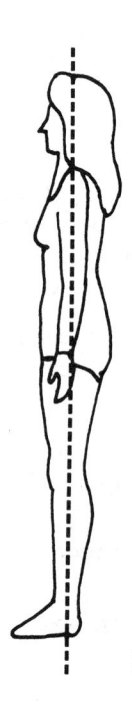

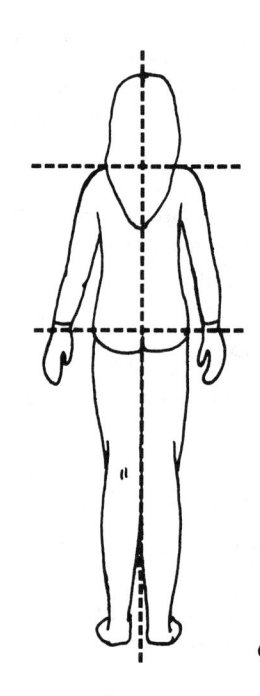

A
B
C

Sitting Posture (D)

1. Alignment of the ear, shoulder and hips.
2. Lower leg flexed—feet drawn in.

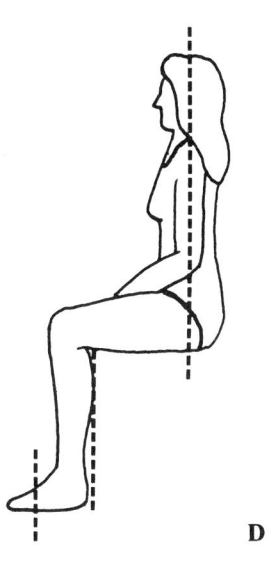

Sleeping Posture (E)

Lying on the side forming S curve is recommended.
1. Sleep on a firm mattress
2. Keep your knees and hips flexed when sleeping on your side

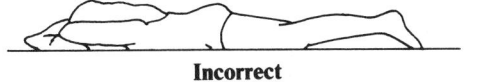

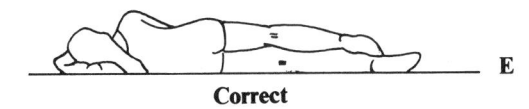

Incorrect

Correct

FUNCTIONAL IMPLICATIONS OF THE LOWER BACK

We should endeavor to make correct posture a habitual form of behavior. Assuming incorrect postures for long periods of time can initiate a number of deviations which result in pain and suffering.

Lower back pain is perhaps one of the most severe complications resulting from poor posture and body mechanics. This debilitating condition usually involves the shortening of a number of muscles of the lower back. This shortening results in stress being placed on the vertebral column and quite often vertebrae are displaced from proper alignment. When vertebrae are not aligned, they tend to press on nerves causing pain in the lower back.

The key in rehabilitation is the removal of stress from the vertebral column. This can be accomplished by removing the cause; i.e., assuming the correct sleeping posture and refraining from lifting resistances beyond our capabilities. In addition, utilization of stretching exercises as a form of therapy and strengthening lower back muscles will relieve this condition.

CARE AND CONSIDERATION OF THE LOWER BACK

Technique of "Walking"

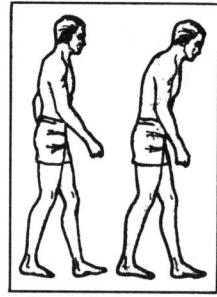

Correct   Incorrect

1. Toe straight ahead when walking. Most of the weight on the heels.
2. Hold chest forward. Elevate the front of the pelvis.
3. Continually try to touch the ceiling with the top of the head.

Mechanics of "Lifting"

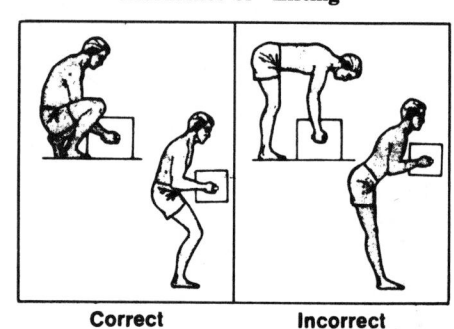

Correct   Incorrect

1. Bend at the knees—squat position.
2. Lift primarily with the thigh muscles, without pressure on the back.
3. *Never* flex forward at the waist with knees straight, attempting to lift with the upper torso.

Skills of "Driving"

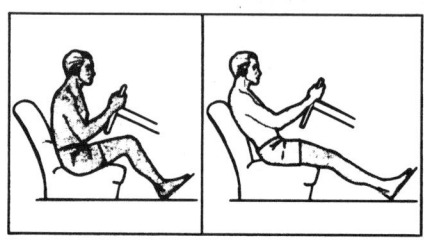

Correct   Incorrect

1. Use a firm seat, with a special seat support, if needed.
2. Sit close to the wheel, with knees bent.
3. Hips back.
4. Stop every two hours, on long trips. Walk and stretch to relax muscles and relieve tension.

Procedure in "Working"

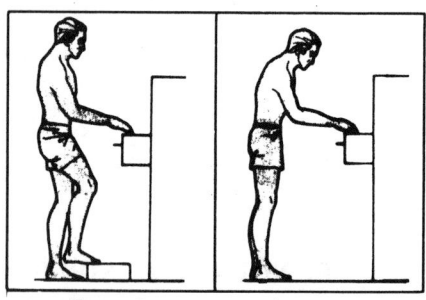

Correct   Incorrect

1. Avoid fatigue caused by work requiring long standing.
2. Flex hips and knees by occasionally placing a foot on a stool or bench.
3. Take exercise breaks from desk work. Move around—perform flexibility and lower back exercises.

Elements of proper body mechanics will follow from these simple maneuvers.

EXERCISE THERAPY FOR THE LOWER BACK

General instructions: The best back support is derived from the muscles of the performance of back exercises often avoids the necessity of using ext€ supports. These supports are usually counter-productive. Back muscles

1. Sissor

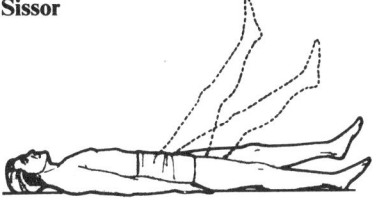

1. Lie in the supine position—legs extended. Arms at the side.
2. Raise legs one at a time, as high as is comfortable—lower leg to the floor as slowly as possible.
3. Repeat five times for each leg, in initial program.

2. Curlup

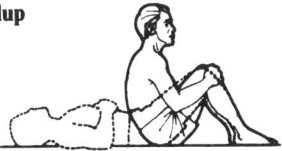

1. Lie in the supine position—knees bent—feet flat on floor.
2. Pull up to a sitting position, keeping knees bent—return to starting position.
3. If necessary have a partner hold your feet down to facilitate this movement.

3. Single Knee Tuck

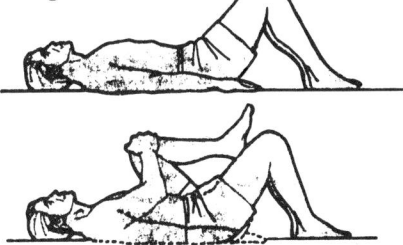

1. Lie in supine position—knees bent—feet flat on the floor.
2. Grasp one knee with both hands and pull close to the chest. Return to starting position.
3. Straighten the leg. Return to starting position.
4. Repeat with alternate leg.

4. Flat-Back

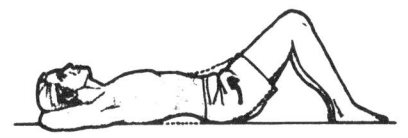

1. Lie in supine position—knees bent, hands clasped behind neck—feet flat on the floor.
2. Press the small of the back against the floor—tighten abdominal and gluteal muscles.
3. Hold for eight seconds—relax.

5. Totem Pole

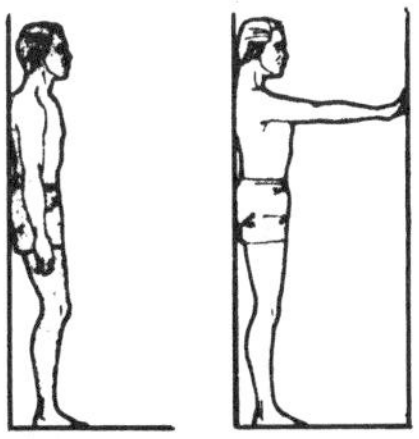

1. Stand with back against doorway.
2. Place heels four inches away from frame.
3. Press the small of back against doorway.
4. Tighten abdominal and gluteal muscles, allowing knees to bend slightly.
5. Now, press neck against doorway, press both hands against opposite side of doorway and straighten both knees.
6. Hold for eight seconds. Relax.

6. Double Knee Tuck

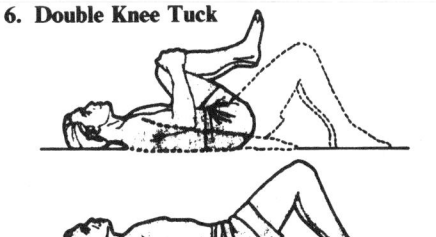

1. Lie in supine position—knees bent.
2. Grasp both knees and pull them close to the chest.
3. Hold for eight seconds—return to starting position.
4. Straighten legs—relax and return to original position.

support needed, if they are strengthened and maintained through regular prescribed exercises.

1. Follow the exercise routine prescribed by your doctor.
2. Gradually increase the frequency of the exercises, as conditioning improves—but stop when fatigued.
3. Wear loose clothing—do not wear shoes.

Selected References

Davies, Evelyn A.: The elementary school child and his posture patterns, Appleton-Century-Crofts, Inc., New York, 1959.
Falls, H. B., Baylor, A. M. and Dishman, R. K. Essentials of fitness. Philadelphia, Saunders College, 1980 p. 74–75.
Kauth, Benjamin: Walk and be happy—a specialists guide to healthy feet. The John Day Company, Inc., New York, 1960.
Tucker, W. E.: Active alerted posture, The Williams & Wilkins Company, Baltimore, 1960.
Wells, K. F., and Luttgens, K.: Kinesiology. Scientific Basis of Human Motion. Philadelphia, W. B. Saunders Co., 1976, p. 151.

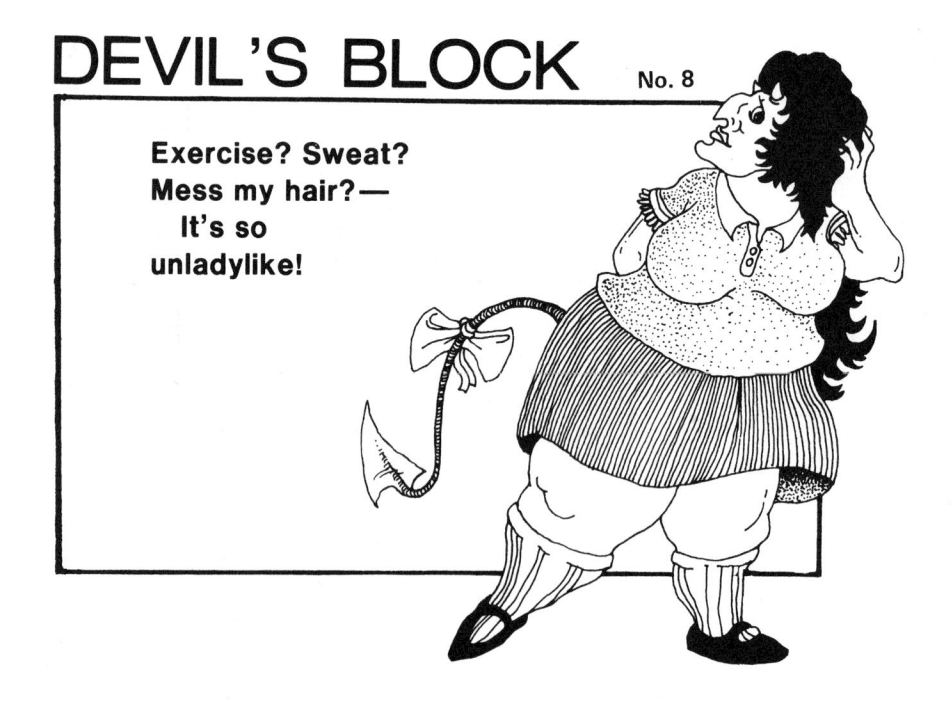

DEVIL'S BLOCK No. 8

Exercise? Sweat? Mess my hair?— It's so unladylike!

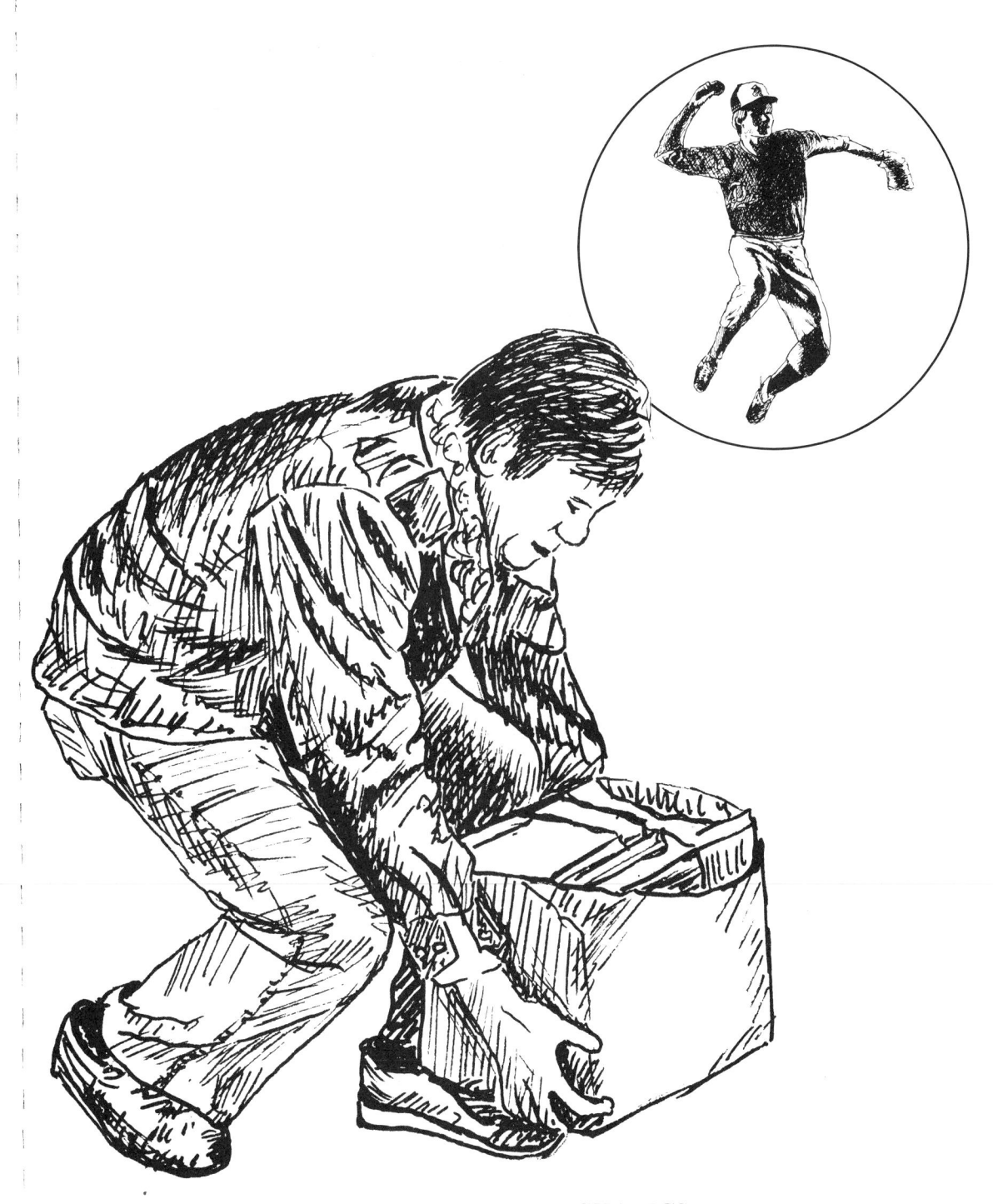

POSTURE AND BODY MECHANICS

PERSONAL APPRAISAL NO. 12
Posture and Body Mechanics

Posture is a state of the human organism that is visible, can be altered, and affects efficient body function. Our purpose in designing this segment is to provide each reader the opportunity of determining present status of one's body position and alignment. You will consider a variety of structural faults and make judgments as to the extent that each can be observed. Although the analysis of each deviation may be somewhat subjective, the test in its entirety will give you a fine indication of your overall state of posture. When interpreting the results, one should recall that deviations are cumulative and, over a long period of time, may gradually increase in severity until structural or permanent damage will result.

Equipment and Facilities
- A. Full-Length Mirror—If Available
- B. Plumb Line

Procedures
- A. Complete this appraisal while working in pairs.
- B. Attire—Bathing Suits
- C. Assume your normal posture in three views (front-side-back) while standing behind a plumb line.
- D. Study the following list of possible postural deviations. Act as the observer while your partner is the subject—then reverse roles. Evaluate each listed deviation and record the score on the five point scale (5 is excellent, deviation not present—1 is extremely poor, deviation is structural (position cannot be changed).

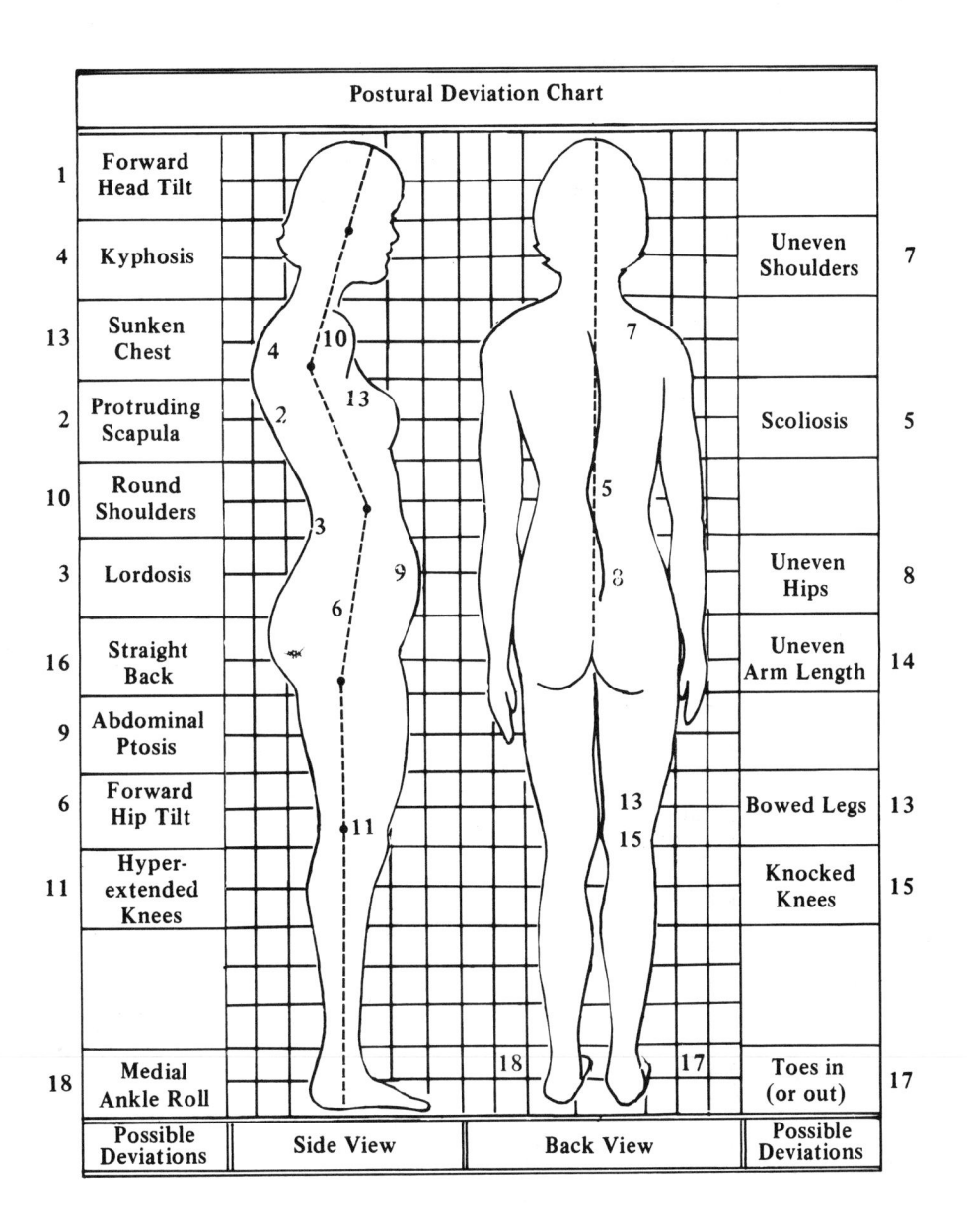

Postural Deviation Chart

Possible Deviations	Side View	Back View	Possible Deviations
1 — Forward Head Tilt			
4 — Kyphosis			7 — Uneven Shoulders
13 — Sunken Chest			
2 — Protruding Scapula			5 — Scoliosis
10 — Round Shoulders			
3 — Lordosis			8 — Uneven Hips
16 — Straight Back			14 — Uneven Arm Length
9 — Abdominal Ptosis			
6 — Forward Hip Tilt			13 — Bowed Legs
11 — Hyperextended Knees			15 — Knocked Knees
18 — Medial Ankle Roll			17 — Toes in (or out)

125

	View	Deviation not Present 5	Deviation Indicated 4	Deviation Visible 3	Deviation Pronounced 2	Deviation Structural (Pos. cannot be Changed) 1	
1. Forward Head Tilt	Side						
2. Protruding Scapula	Side						
3. Lordosis	Side						
4. Kyphosis	Side						
5. Scoliosis	Back						
6. Forward Hip Tilt	Side						
7. Uneven Shoulders	Front						
8. Uneven Hips	Front						
9. Abdominal Ptosis	Side						
10. Round Shoulders	Side						
11. Hyperextended Knees	Side						
12. Bowed Legs	Back						
13. Sunken Chest	Front						
14. Uneven Arm Length	Front						
15. Knocked Knees	Front						
16. Straight Back	Side						
17. Foot (toe in or out)	Back						
18. Medial Ankle Roll	Back						Total Score
	Column Total						

Add each of the vertical columns. Then record the total score.

EVALUATION SHEET
Personal Appraisal No. 12

Name _____

Date _____

Lifetime Participation

I. *Title:* Posture and Body Mechanics

II. *Objectives:*

III. *Results:*

Range of Postural Deviations

Deviation Scores	5	4	3	2	1	Total Score

Scale

	Score	Rating
1	78–90	Excellent Body Posture
2	68–77	Very Good
3	58–67	Good
4	48–57	Fair
5	38–47	Poor
6	28–37	Very Poor
7	18–27	Extremely Poor Posture

IV. *Analysis:*

1. What knowledge concerning your posture did you learn through completing this personal appraisal? Explain.

2. In analyzing your postural deviations, state the possible causes for each deviation.

	Deviation	Cause
a.		
b.		
c.		
d.		
e.		
f.		

3. Has your health been affected by any of your deviations? Yes   No
Explain!

4. Has your ability to engage in physical activity been affected by any of your deviations? Yes   No
Explain!

V. *Implications:*

1. Develop a program of activities designed to improve your posture.

2. Describe the manner in which posture can be a positive influence in life.

NUTRITION—WEIGHT CONTROL

Concepts of Nutrition

Nutrition can be defined as the process of ingesting and assimilating food in promoting growth, providing for metabolism and replacing worn or injured tissue. In short, it is the science of food procurement and usage by the human organism. Its importance in promoting optimal health cannot be underestimated. It has been stated "you are what you eat". This statement holds great truth since diet plays a vital role in mans physiological processes.

The metabolism of the human body requires that a number of substances be consumed each day. These substances which are necessary for the bodies functional maintainance are termed nutrients. A healthful approach to nutrition can be easily achieved since nutrients are found in a wide variety of foods. It is ironic that in our culture a large number of individuals suffer from malnutrition. The reasons for this dichotomy include: poverty, drugs, a lack of knowledge, improper weight loss, lack of will and consumer fraud. Malnutrition could be substantially reduced if individuals possess adequate nutritional information when making dietary decisions.

BASIC NUTRIENTS

Six basic nutrients are necessary for the achievement of a well-balanced diet. These include proteins, carbohydrates, fats, vitamins, minerals and water. Some authorities suggest that roughage be included as a seventh nutrient.

Protein

Except for water, protein is the most abundant substance in human cells. During digestion dietary protein is broken down to the much smaller amino acids. Thirteen non-essential amino acids are synthesized by the human body. Ten others which are not synthesized in the body are termed essential and must be included in the diet. These proteins are found in foods such as meat, milk, poultry, fish, eggs and cheese. Proteins perform a wide variety of functions including; building and repairing tissue, controlling the genetic code, and acting as enzymes. In addition, protein molecules can be utilized as a source of energy when carbohydrate and fat stores are depleted.

Carbohydrates

Carbohydrates are broken down to glucose and glycogen through a series of chemical processes. The major function of carbohydrates in the form of glucose is to provide the body with energy. Glycogen is stored in the liver and muscle tissue to be used as an energy source when glucose levels are insufficient. Fifty percent of the calories ingested are from carbohydrates. The primary source of carbohydrates is in the form of sugars and starches derived from plants.

Fats

Like carbohydrates, fats primary function is that of an energy source. In addition fat is necessary for proper growth, healthy skin and the transportation of fat soluable vitamins. Fats are known as a concentrated source of energy because they have more than twice the energy value of protein and carbohydrates. Fat intake should be monitered since excess fat provides great numbers of calories that will be stored as adipose tissue. Fats are plentiful in liquid vegetable oils, fish oils, meats, butter, cream, whole milk, cheese, egg yolks and nuts.

Vitamins

These are organic substances which are required to perform specific functions. Vitamins are necessary in small quantities. A simple but sound approach is to eat a balanced diet from the basic food groups to insure that appropriate vitamins are present. When a deficiency of a specific vitamin occurs some of the body's cells are unable to function properly and signs indicating a deficiency begin to appear.

Minerals

These inorganic compounds function in growth and repair of tissues and in the regulation of many vital processes. Like vitamins, an inadequacy of mineral intake would result in a deficiency. Calcium, phosphorous, sodium, potassium, magnesium and sulfur are called macro-minerals since we require a generous amount in our diet. Other *trace minerals* necessary in smaller amounts include iron, copper, manganese, iodine, zinc, cobalt, selenium and flourine. Recommended proportions from the basic four food groups more than adequately provide all of the necessary minerals.

Water

Water is the fluid medium of the body and comprises from 40 to 60% of the total body weight. Water is of extreme importance to life and water deprivation for just a few days would result in death. It functions as the bodies fluid medium, in digestion and absorption and in temperature regulation. Water is continually lost by the body therefore it must be constantly replaced. Drinking water is the primary source of this fluid. However, it is also present in a variety of foods including meats, fruits and vegetables.

THE BASIC FOUR FOOD GROUPS

A well-balanced daily diet should include the following four food groups to meet the need for protein, carbohydrates, fats, vitamins, minerals and water.

I Milk Group	II Meat and Protein Group	III Fruit and Vegetable Group	IV Bread and Cheese Group
Includes • Milk • Yogurt • Cottage cheese • Cheese • Other milk products	*Includes:* • Poultry (3 oz.) • Fish (3 oz.) • Eggs (1) • Beef (3 oz.) • Pork (3 oz.) • Lamb (3 oz.) • Dry peas, lentils, beans (1 cup) • Nuts (4 T.)	*Includes:* • Raw fruits (1 medium or 1/2 c., cut up) • Green and yellow vegetables (1/2 c.) • Citrus juice (1/2 c.) • Plus berries, potatoes, etc.	*Includes:* • Whole grain, enriched or restored breads (1 slice) • Pasta (1/2 c.) • Cereal (1 oz.) corn meal, oats • Rice (1/2 c.)
Amount: • 2 One-cup servings (or equivalent) a day	*Amount:* • 2 or more servings a day	*Amount:* • 4 servings a day	*Amount:* • 3–4 servings a day

Choose: Polyunsaturated fats, oils; low-fat, low-sugar desserts.
Avoid: High calorie baked goods, deep-fried foods, cream products, sauces, gravies.

Ideal Body Weight

Body weight is a critical factor that strongly influences our state of condition and health. Body weight has a bearing upon the intensity and type of physical activity in which a person chooses to engage. Conversely, one's involvement in physical activity can play an important role in weight control. A strong relationship exists between body weight, diet, conditioning level, heredity, sex, smoking, and stress tolerance in the prevention of heart and circulatory disorders. Those of us capable of maintaining proper body weight have lowered the risk of developing degenerative heart disease.

Research shows that the death rate for individuals 15–24 percent overweight is 20 percent greater than for individuals who are not overweight but of the same age. An even more striking statistic is a 50 percent greater death rate for men 65 percent overweight. This mortality rate may be the result of the close relationship between being overweight and other degenerative diseases, such as atherosclerosis and high blood pressure.

Ideal weight differs according to our physical characteristics (sex, height, bone structure) and our vocational and recreational interests. Obviously a tall male with large bones and connective tissue will have a greater ideal weight than a person with opposite physical characteristics. Individuals engaged in an occupation or sport such as lumbering, piano moving, or weight-lifting, activities requiring high levels of strength, may need additional muscle mass resulting in increased weight.

People who satisfy nutritional requirements and have acceptable deposits of stored fat are generally more healthy. With lowered body weight, the heart and transport system have less tissue to nourish and therefore have less work to perform. The addition of lean muscle tissue to body weight is acceptable, however, if one gains "fat weight," body effectiveness is decreased. If you are healthy, thin and have muscular tone, you are undoubtedly approaching your ideal weight. The mirror affords the best indication of how close you approach this goal.

Energy Source

The source of fuels which provide energy is primarily fat and carbohydrate. Protein becomes a significant source during starvation. Excess food is stored in fat cells and can be utilized as an energy source when needed. We often measure food in terms of calories. The caloric unit (kilocalorie) is described as the quantity of heat necessary to raise the temperature of one kilogram of water, one degree centigrade. All foods yield varying amounts of calories. A pound of fat will yield 3500 calories. If caloric intake remains the same, and one's exercise expenditure burns an additional 300 calories per day for 12 days, a pound of fat will be lost.

Fundamentals of Weight Control

Weight gain and weight loss are both important considerations. Gaining weight occurs when we overeat, under-exercise or when our metabolic rate decreases. Basal Metabolic rate refers to the minimum energy needed to maintain the normal processes of the body at rest.

Due to a high metabolic rate, some individuals have difficulty gaining weight. High "Force Fed" carbohydrate diets which are often recommended for weight gain are rather disappointing since they provide only 1860 calories per pound, while fat yields 3500 calories per pound. It seems more logical to ingest large amounts of meat containing fat since this provides a significant increase in the calories consumed. Using dietary supplements, regular meals, eating slightly more at each meal than you desire, and snacking also help in promoting a weight gain.

The great majority of weight-conscious people are primarily interested in fat reduction. Divergent points of view exist as to whether dieting or exercise exerts the most pronounced effect on losing weight. Both methods are valuable, and ideally, a combination of the two will bring forth excellent results.

The most dramatic and efficient method of burning fat and losing weight is to eliminate eating. This technique is recommended for brief periods of time (2–5 days). Unfortunately, if dietary habits are not altered, any weight loss will quickly return. A more reasonable method of dieting would be to simply eat less at each meal and eliminate snacks. This will result in a considerable reduction of daily caloric intake. If this intake falls below the bodies metabolic requirements, stored fat will be utilized as an energy source and weight loss will occur. If we eat less, eliminate snacks and reduce carbohydrate and fat intake, our weight loss will be even greater. Simply eating whole wheat bread rather than white bread, low-fat or skim milk rather than whole milk; fish, fowl and lean meats, will exert a positive influence on weight loss.

Becoming physically active results in a speed-up of the metabolic rate causing an increase in the number of calories burned per minute. Contrary to popular belief, this does not necessitate an increase in consumption of food and caloric intake. This heightened metabolic rate may persist for hours after the activity has been concluded. The amount of weight loss is small if viewed on a daily basis, but if one perseveres over a period of time, weight reduction can be substantial. A 150-pound man jogging a twelve-minute mile (5 miles per hour) would burn only 10 calories per minute or 120 calories above normal daily requirements. If continued for a year this routine would result in a 10 1/2 pound weight loss. This is an extremely substantial drop in weight in view of the fact this person initially weighed only 150 pounds. The most practical and healthful method of weight reduction would be to reduce caloric intake and increase daily activity, while maintaining proper nutrition through a well-balanced diet. This procedure would bring forth an efficient loss of weight and a positive effect on total health.

The chart on the following page shows the relationship between the variables effecting weight control: (1) Caloric Intake; (2) Physical Activity; (3) Personal Habits; (4) Metabolic Rate.

Star Factors in Weight Control

The mixture of these factors is constantly changing throughout life. Which path through the maze for weight (fat) control?—*The choice is yours!*

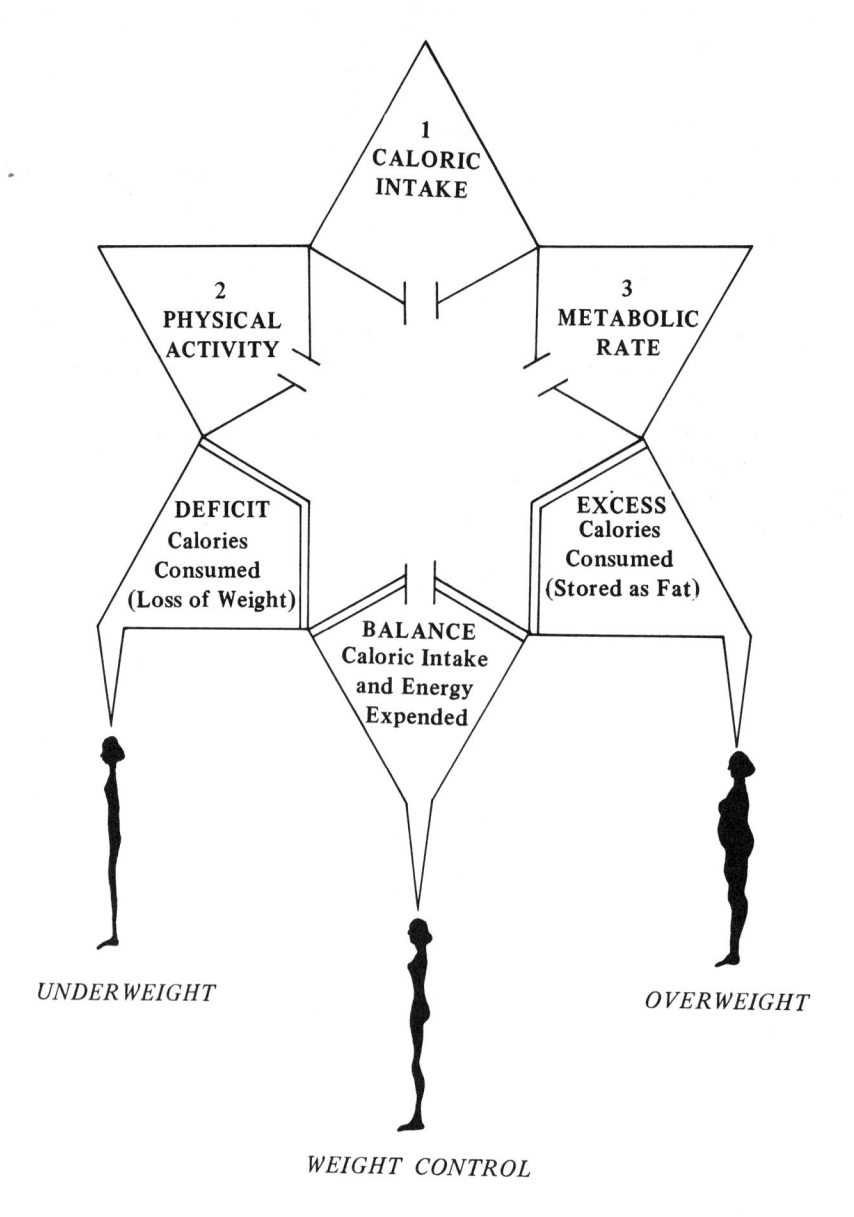

```
              1
           CALORIC
           INTAKE

   2                      3
PHYSICAL              METABOLIC
ACTIVITY                RATE


  DEFICIT               EXCESS
  Calories             Calories
  Consumed             Consumed
(Loss of Weight)     (Stored as Fat)
              BALANCE
           Caloric Intake
            and Energy
             Expended
```

UNDERWEIGHT   OVERWEIGHT

WEIGHT CONTROL

NOTE: Our personal habits are an important factor for success to be realized, as we strive for proper balance between caloric intake, exercise, and metabolic rate. It is extremely important to meet nutritional needs through consumption of a well-balanced diet.

Metabolic rate is the energy required for normal daily functions and body heat.

DIET CONTROL

Diet Control is a very important part of weight control. Goal: To establish perma eating habits that one will maintain throughout life.

General Guidelines to Follow		
1. **Lose Weight Gradually** Weight loss should average only a few pounds per week.	**2.** **Space Meals Evenly** Keep meals approximately the same size and space evenly throughout the day.	**3.** **Don't Skip Meals** Irregular meals make fattening snacks more tempting.
4. **Eat Slowly** Chew each mouthful thoroughly. Primary digestion takes place here. Put down your fork frequently. Stop eating when you feel full.	**5.** **Plan Snacks** Save part of your caloric allowance to snack on later, instead of going on fad diets or fasts.	**6.** **Watch Your Progress** Weigh yourself once a week, at the same time of the day.

TIPS FOR THE SUCCESSFUL DIET

1. Keep a list of everything you eat or drink. Keep a notebook handy and record what you eat, the amount and time you consumed it.
2. Eliminate sugar from your diet.
3. Avoid high sugar (carbohydrate foods) such as candy, pastries, fruit juice with sugar, sugar coated cereals, ice cream cakes, pies and soft drinks.
4. Find acceptable snacktime substitutes for the above. Fruits, carrots, celery, etc. are excellent.
5. Use only vegetable oils for cooking. Use these sparingly.
6. Trim fat from meats. Use lean meats exclusively.
7. Decrease use of butter and margarines to no more than 3 patties per day.
8. Eat your favorite raw vegetables in any quantity desired. These are low calorie foods which are high in nutrients.
9. Avoid highly seasoned foods.
10. Consume low calorie foods such as unsweetened tea and coffee, clear broth, unsweetened lemon, pickles and gelatin, and fat free bouillon.
11. Restrict eating during periods of emotional upset.
12. Take small helpings and avoid second helpings.
13. Do not store high calorie and empty calorie foods at home. Reduce temptation.
14. Drink a liberal amount of water each day.

Selected References

Borgstrom, B. Lipid absorption—Physiochemical considerations. In J. Wakil (Ed.), Metabolism and physiological significance of Lipids. New York: Academic Press, 1970.

Katch, F. I., and McArdle, W. D. Nutrition, weight control and exercise. Boston: Houghton-Mifflin, 1977.

Keys, A., Fidanza, F., Karvonen, M. J., Kimura, N., and Taylor, H. I. Indicies of relative weight and obesity. *Journal of Chronic Diseases,* 1972, 25, 329–343.

Patrizkova, J. Body fat and physical fitness. The Hague: Martinus Nijhoff, 1977.

Soloni, F. G. Determination of blood trigliceride levels. *Clinical Chemistry,* 1971, 171, 529.

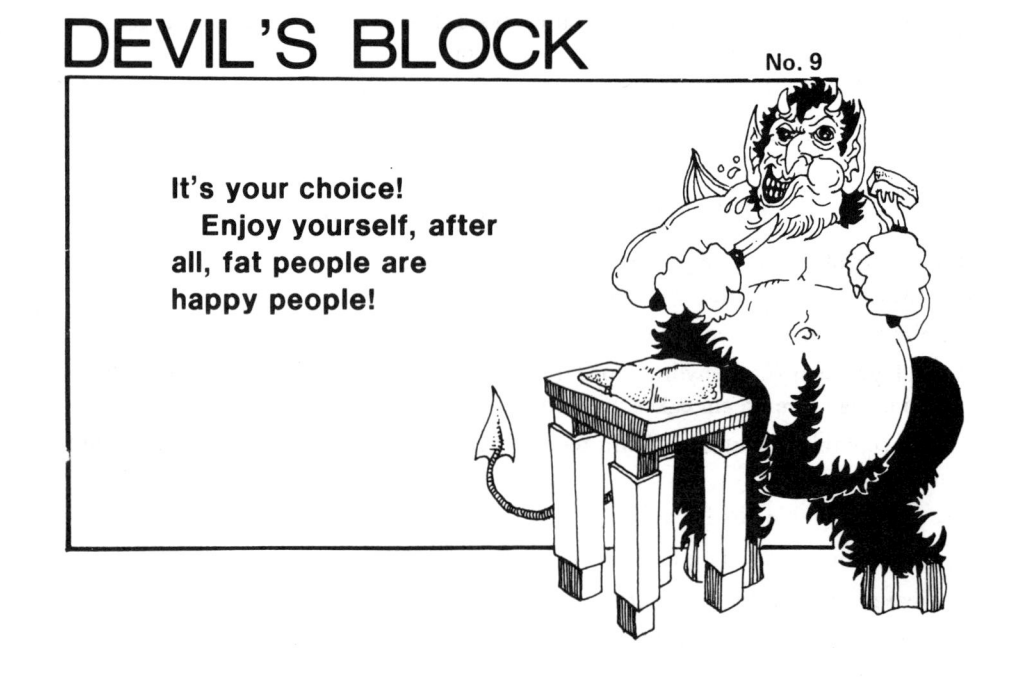

DEVIL'S BLOCK — No. 9

It's your choice! Enjoy yourself, after all, fat people are happy people!

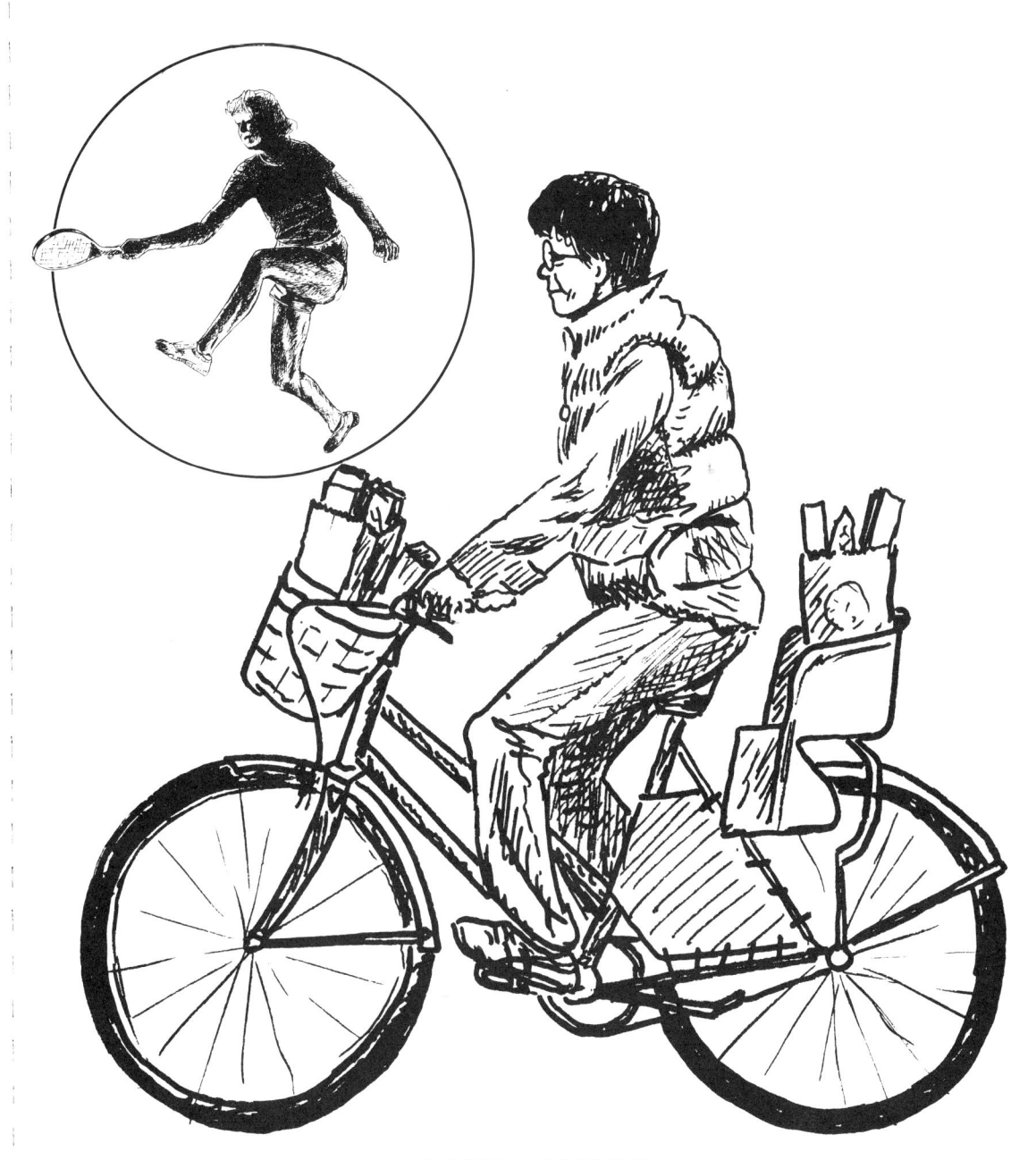

WEIGHT CONTROL

PERSONAL APPRAISAL NO 13
Obesity

Obesity can be defined as a condition in which the body has excess deposits of stored fat. The simple phrase "too much fat" concisely describes this condition. Although most obese people are overweight, all overweight people are not necessarily obese. Overweight occurs in some individuals as a result of large bones and muscle mass or excessive accumulation of tissue fluid, but without excessive fatness.

Obesity is a serious problem not only for adults but for millions of American teenagers. Studies of this age group have resulted in clues which indicate the emergence of the under-exercise obese cycle. Research has shown that youngsters gain weight not because they eat more than their more slender schoolmates, but because they exercise so little. A vicious cycle begins as the youngster becomes heavier, less energy is expended. They become extremely bashful to join in physical activity, and this cycle soon becomes a permanent part of their lives. Physical inactivity is the single most important factor explaining the increasing frequency of overweight people in our society.

The use of height and weight tables in assessing obesity is often misleading. Standard height and weight tables do not take into account the extent of muscle tissue. Football players who have developed large areas of muscle mass usually rate poorly on these tables; however, the percent of their total body weight comprised of fat may be minimal. Intensive physical conditioning can cause a depletion of excess fat and an increase in lean muscle tissue with no appreciable change in body weight.

Approximately 50 percent of the body's fat is stored subcutaneously or just below the skin. One method of evaluating body fat is to measure skinfold thickness. This is accomplished with the use of skinfold calipers. However, an extremely simple yet effective technique is to pinch the skin between the thumb and index finger. If the resulting mass is thicker than one inch, obesity is indicated. If this occurs in more than one area of the body, there is an even greater indication of obesity.

Facilities and Equipment

    A. Skinfold Calipers

Procedures

A. Take the following measurements—using skinfold calipers.

1. Men
   a. Triceps—taken at the mid-point between the elbow and the shoulder of the dominant arm.
   b. Chest—slightly above and to the outside of the right nipple.
   c. Navel—taken at the mid-point between the navel and the right side of the body—use a vertical fold.
2. Women
   a. Triceps—same as above.
   b. Navel—same as above.
   c. Iliac crest—taken 1″ above the iliac crest, on the right side—use a horizontal fold.

B. Grasp skin between the thumb and index finger in a manner that allows you to differentiate the separation of skin and fat layers from muscle tissue. When performed correctly, only the layers of skin and subcutaneous fat deposits will be measured.

EVALUATION SHEET
Personal Appraisal No. 13

Name _____

Date _____

Lifetime Participation

  I. *Title:* Obesity

 II. *Objective:*

III. *Results:*

Record your score from 1 to 3 for each skinfold measurement in the appropriate block at the bottom of each column and total.

Skinfold Thickness Measurements	
_____	Tricep
_____	Navel
_____	Chest
_____	Iliac Crest

	Skinfold Thickness Scale						
	Point Rating	Female			Male		
		Triceps	Navel	Iliac Crest	Triceps	Navel	Chest
Overfatness not Indicated	1	0-14	0-12	0-10	0-11	0-9	0-8
Overfatness Indicated	2	15-28	13-26	11-25	12-24	10-21	9-20
Gross Overfatness Indicated	3	29+	27+	26+	25+	22+	21+
Score Rating 1 to 3							
		Total Score			Total Score		

Obesity Scale	
Total Score 3—Excellent 4—Good 5-6—Fair 7-8—Poor 9—Very poor	Nonobese ↑ ↓ Obese

IV. *Analysis:*

1. Do the results of this appraisal substantiate or contradict your perceptions of your body weight held prior to taking this test? Explain!

2. State your present body weight _____ lbs. and what you feel should be your ideal body weight _____ lbs. Explain the reason for any difference.

3. Relate any experiences that you have had in which an altered body weight would have been to your advantage.

V. *Implications:*

1. Describe the changes in life style necessary to correct the difference between your present body weight and your ideal body weight.

PERSONAL APPRAISAL NO. 14
Body Weight and Caloric Balance

The purpose of this appraisal is to examine the factors involved with caloric intake and output and to determine the extent to which the amount of calories you consume and the amount of calories you metabolise effects your body weight. When the number of calories injested is equal to the number of calories burned, body weight remains stable. When this caloric balance shifts to either side of the fulcrum, a weight loss or weight gain occurs. To underscore this delicate balance, imagine caloric intake exceeding caloric output by 200 Kcal per day. In a year, the individual will have injested an additional 73,000 Kcal or 20.8 lbs., (365 days × 200 Kcal = 73,000 Kcal v 3,500 = 20.8). This weight gain would occur if one were to drink an additional 16 ounces of beer each day for one year without a corresponding increase in exercise.

We can determine the number of calories consumed in an average day by keeping a detailed chart of all the foods consumed during a specific period of time. We can also compute the approximate number of calories burned during this same time period. By comparing these two figures, we are able to project an idea of the state of our caloric balance.

Considerations:

    A. Metabolism is affected by:
        1. Body weight
        2. Age
        3. Sex
        4. Physical condition

    B. Metabolizing one pound of stored fat is the equivalent of burning 3,500 Kcal.

Facilities and Equipment:

    A. Physical activity energy expenditure chart

    B. Caloric value food chart

Procedures:

A. Use the caloric value food chart on page 147 to complete the five-day caloric intake assessment (Page 145). Total caloric column 1, 2, 3, and 4, and record at bottom. Add these four figures to determine the five-day total caloric intake. Divide the total number of calories for five days by five. This results in your average daily caloric intake total. Record Tuesday through Saturday or Sunday through Thursday.

B. Use the physical activity energy expenditure chart on page 157 to fill in the five day physical activity chart. (Page 146). Divide the total number of calories burned for five days by five. This results in your average caloric output per day.

C. Determine the difference between your average daily caloric intake and your average daily caloric output.

Caloric Intake Assessment									
Five Consecutive Days	Column 1			Column 2		Column 3		Column 4	
	Breakfast Food	1 Cal.	Lunch Food	2 Cal.	Dinner Food	3 Cal.	Snack Food	4 Cal.
1								
2								
3								
4								
5								
	Column 1 Total _____		Column 2 Total _____		Column 3 Total _____		Column 4 Total _____	

Grand total-caloric intake five days = _____

Divide grand total by five = Average daily Caloric intake _____

	Daily Physical Activity Chart							
Five Consecutive Days	Column A		Column B		Column C		Column D	
	Morning 8 A.M.-1 P.M.	Cal. Burn	Afternoon 1 P.M.-6 P.M.	Cal. Burn	Evening 6 P.M.-10 P.M.	Cal. Burn	Night 10 P.M.-8 A.M.	Cal. Burn
1								
2								
3								
4								
5								
	Column A Total _____		Column B Total _____		Column C Total _____		Column D Total _____	
Energy expended Grand total _____		Divide grand total by five		=		Average daily Caloric output _____	

I
Nutrition and Calorie Chart

Food	Weight Gm.	Calories	Protein Gm.	Fat Gm.	Carbohydrate Gm.
Alcoholic beverages					
beer, 12 oz. glass	360	150	NA	NA	13.7
whiskey, rum, gin, vodka, etc.					
100 proof, 1 1/2 oz. gigger	42	124	NA	NA	TR
90 proof, 1 1/2 oz. gigger	42	110	NA	NA	TR
80 proof, 1 1/2 oz. gigger	42	95	NA	NA	TR
wine (dessert) 3 1/2 oz. glass	103	140	.1	0	7.8
wine (table) 3 1/2 oz. glass	102	86	.1	0	4.3
Almonds, roasted, shelled 1/2 cup	78	486	14.4	45.0	15.0
Apples, raw whole 1 lb.	150	70	18	TR	TR
Apple juice, 1/2 cup	124	60	15	TR	TR
Applesauce, canned, sweetened, 1 cup	255	230	.5	.3	60.7
Apricot nectar, canned 6 oz. glass	188	105	.6	.2	27.4
apricots, raw 1 average (about 12/lb.)	38	15	.4	TR	4.5
Asparagus, canned spears, drained, 1 cup	215	43	5.2	.9	7.3
Bacon, cooked crisp, drained, 2 slices	15	90	4.5	7.8	.5
bacon, Canadian, cooked crisp, drained, 1 slice	15	40	4.1	2.6	TR
Bagal, water, 1 medium (3" diameter)	55	163	6.0	2.0	30.0
Bananas, peeled, 1 medium	119	100	1.3	.2	26.4
Barbecue sauce, 1 cup	250	225	3.7	17.2	20.0
Bass, sea, raw, 4 oz.	114	115	21.9	1.4	0
Bean sprouts, mung, raw, 1 cup	90	32	3.4	.2	6.0
Baked beans, canned, in tomato sauce, 8 oz.	227	270	14.3	1.1	52.2
baked beans w/frankfurters, 8 oz.	227	325	17.3	16.1	28.6
Beans, green or snap, raw, whole, 1 lb.	454	125	7.6	.8	28.3
beans, lima, raw, immature, in pods, 1 lb.	454	221	15.2	.9	40.1
Beef, choice grade, retail trim, meat only, 4 oz:					
chuck, boneless arm, pot roasted, lean & fat	114	326	30.9	21.8	0
chuck, boneless arm, pot roasted, lean only	114	218	34.9	7.9	0
club steak, broiled, lean & fat	114	515	23.0	46.3	0
club steak, broiled, lean only	114	278	33.7	14.8	0
flank stead, pot roasted	114	220	34.8	8.3	0
ground, regular, broiled	114	324	27.6	23.1	0
porterhouse steak broiled, lean & fat	114	527	22.4	48.1	0
rib roasted, lean & fat	114	500	22.7	43.9	0
round, broiled, lean & fat	114	295	32.6	17.5	0
rump, roasted, lean & fat	114	392	26.9	31.1	0
sirloin steak, double bone, broiled, lean & fat	114	463	25.3	39.5	0
sirloin steak, double bone, broiled, lean only	114	243	34.8	10.8	0
sirloin steak, round bone, broiled, lean & fat	114	440	26.2	36.5	0
T-bone steak, broiled, lean & fat	114	536	22.2	49.2	0
T-bone, lean only	114	252	34.6	11.7	0
Beef, corned, boiled, medium fat, 4 oz.	114	422	26.1	34.6	0
canned, medium fat, 4 oz.	114	243	28.7	13.6	0
Beef, dried or chipped, uncooked, 4 oz.	114	230	39.1	6.2	0
Beef pot pie, frozen, 8 oz. pie	227	433	16.6	22.5	40.9
Beef roast, canned, 4 oz.	114	252	28.3	14.8	0
Beet greens, boiled, drained, 1 cup	200	35	3.4	.4	6.6
Blackberries, fresh, 1 cup	146	83	1.8	1.3	18.8
Blueberries, fresh, 1 cup	146	88	1.2	.4	35.6
blueberries, frozen, sweetened, 1 cup	228	236	1.4	.7	60.4
blueberries, unsweetened, 1 cup	165	90	1.2	.8	22.4
Bluefish, baked or broiled w/butter, 4 oz.	114	180	29.9	5.9	0

Food	Weight Gm.	Calories	Protein Gm.	Fat Gm.	Carbohydrate Gm.
Bologna, all meat, 4 oz.	114	310	14.9	25.6	4.2
Bouillon cube, 1/2 cube	4	5	.8	.1	.2
Bread, French or Vienna, 1 slice, 3/4" x 2" x 1"	20	55	1.8	.6	11.1
bread, Italian, 1 slice, 3 1/4" x 2" x 1"	20	53	1.8	.1	11.3
bread, pumpernickel, 1 slice, 3 3/4" x 3 3/4" x 1/8"	30	72	2.7	.4	15.9
bread, raisin, 1 slice	23	58	1.5	.6	12.3
bread, rye, light, 1 slice	23	55	2.1	.2	11.9
bread, white, 1 slice	23	60	2.0	.7	11.6
bread, whole wheat, 1 slice	23	54	2.4	.7	11.0
bread, white, 1 thin slice	17	45	1.5	.5	8.6
Bread stuffing mix, dry, 1 cup	71	260	9.1	2.7	51.4
Brocoli, fresh, cuts, boiled, drained, 1 cup	155	38	4.8	.5	7.0
Brussels sprouts, fresh, boiled, drained, 1 cup	180	63	7.6	.7	11.5
Butter, 1 tablespoon	14	98	.1	11.3	TR
butter, whipped, 1 tablespoon	9	62	.1	7.3	TR
Cabbage, common, shredded, boiled, drained, 1 cup	145	29	1.6	.3	6.2
cabbage, Chinese, raw, 1" cuts, 1 cup	75	11	9	.1	2.2
Cake mixes, prepared, 4 oz. piece:					
angel food, prepared w/water, flavoring	114	293	6.5	.2	67.7
chocolate malt (w/eggs) water, icing	114	392	3.9	9.9	75.9
coffeecake (w/eggs), milk	114	365	7.2	10.9	59.7
devil's food (w/eggs), water, icing	114	383	5.0	14.0	66.5
gingerbread, prepared w/water	114	313	3.5	7.8	58.2
marble (w/eggs), water, icing	114	375	5.0	9.9	70.7
white (w/egg whites), water, icing	114	397	4.4	12.2	71.6
yellow (w/eggs), water, icing	114	382	4.7	12.9	65.7
Cake, devil's food, frozen, w/icing	114	430	4.9	20.1	63.4
Candies, 1 oz.:					
almonds, chocolate coated	28	159	3.5	12.4	11.2
almonds, sugar coated	28	127	2.2	5.3	19.9
butterscotch	28	110	TR	1.0	26.9
caramel, plain or chocolate	28	111	1.1	2.9	21.7
carmel, plain or chocolate w/nuts	28	120	1.3	4.6	20.0
chocolate, milk	28	145	2.2	9.2	16.1
chocolate, milk, w/almonds	28	149	2.6	10.1	14.5
chocolate, milk, w/peanuts	28	152	4.0	10.8	12.6
chocolate, milk, sugar coated	28	130	1.5	5.6	20.6
chocolate, sweet	28	145	1.2	9.9	16.4
chocolate fudge, chocolate coated	28	120	1.1	4.5	20.7
chocolate fudge w/nuts, chocolate coated	28	125	1.4	5.9	19.0
fudge, vanilla	28	111	.9	3.1	21.2
hard candy	28	107	0	.3	27.6
jelly beans	28	104	TR	.1	26.4
marshmallows	28	88	.6	TR	22.8
peanuts, chocolate coated	28	157	4.6	11.7	11.1
raisins, chocolate coated	28	118	1.5	4.8	20.0
Cantaloupe, 1/2 melon (5" diameter)	385	56	1.4	.2	14.5
Carrots, raw, 1 medium (5 1/2" x 1")	50	20	.5	.1	4.8
carrots, raw, grated or shredded, 1 cup	109	45	1.2	.2	10.6
Cashew nuts, roasted, shelled, 4 oz.	114	635	19.6	52.1	33.4
Catsup, tomato, bottled, 1 tablespoon	17	16	.3	TR	4.3
Cauliflower, boiled, drained, 1 cup	125	26	2.9	.3	5.1
cauliflower, frozen, boiled, drained, 1 cup	179	30	3.4	.4	5.9
Celery, raw, 1 outer stalk (8" long)	40	6	.4	TR	1.6
celery, raw, chopped or diced, 1 cup	119	18	1.1	.1	4.6

Food	Weight Gm.	Calories	Protein Gm.	Fat Gm.	Carbohydrate Gm.
Cereal, ready-to-eat, bran flakes, 40%, 1 oz.	28	85	2.9	.5	22.8
bran flakes, w/raisins, 1 oz.	28	80	2.3	.4	22.5
corn, puffed, presweetened, 1 oz.	28	105	1.1	TR	25.4
corn flakes	28	107	2.2	.1	24.2
corn flakes, sugar coated, 1 oz.	28	107	1.2	TR	25.9
oats, puffed, 1 oz.	28	110	3.4	1.6	21.3
oats, puffed, sugar coated, 1 oz.	28	109	1.9	1.0	24.3
rice, puffed, 1 oz.	28	111	1.7	.1	25.4
rice, shredded, 1 oz.	28	109	1.5	.1	25.2
wheat, puffed, 1 oz.	28	102	4.2	.4	22.3
wheat, shredded, 1 oz.	28	98	2.6	.6	22.6
wheat flakes, 1 oz.	28	98	2.7	.4	22.8
oatmeal	20	76	2.8	1.5	13.6
Cheese, American, processed, 1 oz.	28	103	6.6	8.5	.5
cheese, American, processed, shredded, 1 cup	111	409	25.8	33.3	2.1
blue or bleu, 1 oz.	28	102	6.1	8.6	.6
cheddar, 1 oz.	28	111	7.1	9.1	.6
cottage cheese, creamed, 1 oz.	28	28	3.8	1.2	.8
cottage cheese, creamed, 1 cup	245	258	33.3	10.3	7.1
cottage cheese, uncreamed, 1 oz.	28	22	4.8	.1	.8
cottage cheese, uncreamed, 1 cup	200	170	34.0	.6	5.4
cream, 1 tablespoon	15	54	1.2	5.6	.3
parmesan cheese, grated, 1 tablespoon	7	26	2.5	1.8	.2
roquefort cheese, 1 oz.	28	102	6.1	8.6	.6
swiss cheese, processed, 1 oz.	28	100	7.5	7.6	.5
Cheese food, American, processed, 1 oz.	28	90	5.6	6.8	2.0
Cherries, red sour, fresh w/pits, 1 cup	160	90	1.9	.5	22.9
cherries, red sour, frozen, sweetened, 4 oz.	114	126	1.1	.5	15.3
cherries, sweet, fresh, w/pits, 1 cup	160	110	2.1	.5	27.8
cherries, candied, 1 oz.	28	94	.1	.1	24.6
Chewing gum, sweetened, 1 ave. stock	3	8	NA	NA	2.8
Chicken, fresh, boiled, meat only, 4 oz.	114	155	27.1	4.3	8
chicken, fried, 1/2 breast w/bone, 3.3 oz.	94	152	24.8	5.0	1.0
chicken, fried, drumstick w/bone, 2.1 oz.	59	87	11.8	4.0	TR
chicken, roasted, dark meat, 4 oz.	114	208	33.4	7.4	0
chicken, roasted, white meat, 4 oz.	114	205	36.8	5.6	0
Chicken pot pie, forzen, 8 oz. pie	227	495	15.2	26.1	50.4
Chili con carne, canned, w/beans, 8 oz.	227	300	17.0	13.8	27.7
chili con carne, canned, no beans, 8 oz.	227	452	23.4	33.6	13.2
Chili sauce, tomato, bottled, 1 tablespoon	16	15	.4	TR	4.0
Chocolate, baking-type, bitter, unsweetened, 1 oz.	28	140	3.0	15.0	8.2
Chocolate syrup, fudge type, 1 tablespoon	20	65	1.0	2.7	10.8
Chocolate syrup, thin type, 1 tablespoon	20	48	15	.4	12.5
Chow mein, chicken, canned, 8 oz.	227	84	5.9	.2	16.1
Clams, hard or round, raw, meat only, 8 oz.	227	180	25.2	2.0	13.4
Cocoa, high fat, processed, 1 tablespoon powder	6	16	1.0	1.4	2.7
cocoa mix, w/nonfat dry milk, 1 tablespoon powder	9	30	1.7	.2	6.4
Coconut, fresh, meat only, 4 oz.	114	390	4.0	40.0	10.7
Cod, fresh, raw, 4 oz.	114	86	19.9	.3	0
cod, fresh, broiled w/butter, 4 oz.	114	192	32.5	6.0	0
cod, frozen, cakes, reheated, 4 oz.	114	306	10.5	20.4	19.6
cod, frozen, fillets, 4 oz. (w ave. fillets)	114	82	18.8	.4	0
cod, frozen, sticks, 4 oz. (5 ave. sticks)	114	275	15.1	10.7	29.1
Coffee, instant, dry, 1 teaspoon	2	2	TR	TR	.7
Coleslaw, commercial, w/French dressing, 4 oz.	114	106	1.4	8.3	8.7

Food	Weight Gm.	Calories	Protein Gm.	Fat Gm.	Carbohydrate Gm.
Cookies, commercial packaged:					
animal crackers, 1 oz.	28	120	1.9	2.7	22.7
assorted, 1 oz.	28	134	1.4	5.7	20.1
brownies, w/nuts, iced, frozen, 1 oz.	28	116	1.4	5.8	17.2
butter, thin, rich, 1 oz.	28	127	1.7	4.8	20.1
chocolate, 1 oz.	28	124	2.0	4.5	20.3
chocolate chip, 1 oz.	28	132	1.5	5.9	19.8
coconut bar, 1 oz.	28	137	1.8	6.9	18.1
fig bar, 1 oz.	28	100	1.1	1.6	21.4
graham crackers, 1 oz.	28	107	2.3	2.7	20.8
graham crackers, chocolate coated, 1 oz.	28	133	1.4	6.7	19.2
ladyfingers, 1 oz.	28	100	2.2	2.2	18.3
marshmallow, 1 oz.	28	114	1.1	3.7	20.5
oatmeal, w/raisins, 1 oz.	28	120	1.8	4.4	20.8
peanut, 1 oz.	28	132	2.8	5.4	19.0
raisin, 1 oz.	28	105	1.2	1.5	22.9
Cookies, baked from mix:					
brownies made w/nuts, 1 oz.	28	112	1.4	5.3	16.9
brownies (w/egg), nuts, 1 oz.	28	119	1.4	5.7	17.9
Corn, sweet, fresh, on cob, boiled, drained, 1 ear (5")	140	70	2.6	.8	16.4
corn, fresh, kernels, boiled, drained, 1 cup	166	135	5.2	1.6	31.2
corn, canned, kernels, boiled, drained, 1 cup	173	142	4.5	1.4	34.3
corn, canned, cream style, 1 cup	253	205	5.3	1.5	50.6
Corn bread mix (w/egg), milk, 2 oz.	57	130	3.6	4.8	18.7
Corn grits, degermed, dry, 1/4 cup	40	142	3.5	.3	31.2
Corn muffin, baked from mix (w/egg), milk, 2 oz.	57	182	3.9	6.0	28.5
Crab, fresh, steamed in shell, 1 lb.	454	200	37.7	4.1	1.1
crab, fresh, steamed, meat only, 4 oz.	114	102	19.6	2.2	.6
Crackers, commercial packaged:					
crackers, barbecue flavor, 1 oz.	28	140	1.9	7.5	18.0
crackers, cheese, 1 oz.	28	133	3.2	6.0	17.1
crackers, peanut butter-cheese sand., 1 oz.	28	137	4.3	6.8	15.9
crackers, saltines, 1 oz.	28	121	2.6	3.4	20.3
Cranberries, fresh, whole, 1 lb.	454	198	1.7	3.0	47.0
Cranberry sauce, canned, sweet, strained, 1 cup	271	396	.3	.5	101.6
Cream, dairy, half & half, 1 cup	242	322	7.7	28.3	11.1
cream, half & half, 1 tablespoon	15	20	.5	1.8	.7
cream, light, table or coffee, 1 tablespoon	15	30	.4	3.1	.6
cream, whipping, light, 1 cup unwhipped	239	715	6.0	74.8	8.6
cream, sour, 1 tablespoon	12	25	.3	2.0	1.0
Cucumber, fresh, w/skin, 1 med., 7 1/2" x 2"	207	30	1.2	.2	6.9
Dates, domestic, natural & dry:					
with pits, 4 oz.	114	268	2.2	.5	71.9
pitted, 4 oz.	114	309	2.5	.6	82.7
Doughnuts, cake type, 1 oz.	28	109	1.3	5.3	14.6
doughnuts, cake type, 1 average	32	122	1.5	5.9	16.4
doughnuts, yeast-leavened, 1 oz.	28	115	1.8	7.7	10.7
Duck, domestic, roasted, meat only, 4 oz.	114	350	75.8	26.7	0
Eggs, chicken, raw, whole, 1 large	50	80	6.4	5.7	.4
egg, boiled, 1 large	50	80	6.4	5.7	.4
egg, poached, 1 large	50	80	6.3	5.8	.4
Eggnog, dairy packaged, 6% butterfat, 1 cup	250	157	4.1	8.3	17.3
Eggplant, raw, whole, 1 lb.	454	90	4.4	.7	20.6
Fishcakes, breaded, frozen, cooked, 4 oz.	114	306	10.5	20.4	19.6
Fish sticks, breaded, frozen, cooked, 4 oz.	114	200	18.7	10.1	7.1

Food	Weight Gm.	Calories	Protein Gm.	Fat Gm.	Carbohydrate Gm.
Flouder, raw, whole, 1 lb.	454	115	25.0	1.2	0
flounder, raw, fillets, 4 oz.	114	88	18.9	.9	0
Frankfurters, raw, average, all, 4 oz.	114	347	14.2	31.3	2.0
frankfurters, raw, all meat, 4 oz.	114	335	14.9	28.9	2.8
Fruit cocktail, canned, w/heavy syrup, 8 oz.	227	170	.9	.3	44.7
Fruit, mixed, frozen, sweetened, 8 oz.	227	248	1.0	.2	63.8
Gelatin, unflavored, dry, 1 package	7	25	6.0	TR	0
unflavored, dry, 1 tablespoon	10	32	8.4	TR	0
flavored, dessert mix, dry, 3 oz. pkg.	85	312	8.0	0	74.6
flavored dessert mix, made w/water, 1 cup	240	140	4.0	0	33.6
Goose, roasted, meat only, 4 oz.	114	264	38.4	11.0	0
Grapefruit, fresh, pink or red, 1/2 medium	284	58	.7	.1	15.0
pink or red, sections, 1 cup	200	80	1.0	.2	20.6
canned, in syrup, 1 cup	256	178	1.4	.3	45.4
Grapefruit juice, fresh, 6 oz. glass	185	78	.8	.1	16.8
canned, sweetened, 6 oz. glass	188	98	.8	.1	24.0
canned, unsweetened, 6 oz. glass	184	76	.8	.1	18.0
frozen, sweetened, diluted, 6 oz. glass	174	80	.7	.2	19.5
Grape juice, canned, 6 oz. glass	185	120	.4	TR	30.5
frozen, sweetened, diluted, 6 oz. glass	185	98	.4	TR	24.4
Grapes, American type, fresh, 1 lb.	450	196	3.5	2.9	44.8
fresh, whole, 1 cup	153	65	1.2	1.0	15.0
Haddock, raw, meat, 4 oz.	114	90	20.6	.1	0
fresh, fillet, breaded, fried, 3 1/2 oz.	100	164	19.5	6.6	5.7
Halibut, Atlantic or Pacific, broiled w/butter, 4 oz.	114	196	28.7	8.0	0
frozen, steak, 4 oz.	114	142	21.0	6.0	0
Ham (meat only), boiled, 4 oz.	114	268	21.6	19.2	0
fresh, medium fat, roasted, 4 oz.	114	424	26.0	34.6	0
Ham, deviled, canned, 2 oz.	57	202	7.6	18.2	0
Ham, spiced, canned, 2 oz.	57	169	8.4	14.1	.7
Herring, Atlantic, raw, meat only, 4 oz.	114	200	19.4	12.7	0
Honey, strained or extracted, 1 tablespoon	21	64	TR	0	17.3
Ice cream and frozen custard:					
regular, approx. 10% fat, 1 cup	133	256	6.0	14.0	27.5
rich, approx. 16% fat, 1 cup	147	328	3.8	23.6	26.6
Ice cream cone, 1 average	5	19	.5	.1	3.7
Ice milk, hardened, 1 cup	130	200	6.3	6.6	29.3
Ices, water, lime, 1 cup	180	140	.6	TR	58.5
Jams and preserves, all flavors, 1 tablespoon	20	52	.1	TR	14.0
Jellies, all flavors, 1 tablespoon	20	54	TR	TR	14.2
Lamb, fresh, choice grade:					
chop, loin, 4.8 oz., broiled, with bone	112	400	24.4	32.9	0
leg, roasted, lean and fat, 4 oz.	114	317	28.6	21.6	0
Lard, 1 tablespoon	13	116	0	13.0	0
Lemonade, frozen, sweetened, diluted, 1 cup	242	105	.2	TR	27.5
Lemon juice, unsweetened:					
fresh, 1/2 cup	123	31	.6	.2	9.7
Lemons, 1 average	110	20	.8	.2	5.8
Lentils, whole, dry, 1 cup	190	644	46.8	2.1	114.0
whole, cooked, drained, 1 cup	200	214	15.7	TR	39.0
Lettuce, iceberg, 1 lb. head	452	58	3.8	.4	12.4
Lime juice, fresh, unsweetened, 1 tablespoon	15	4	TR	TR	1.4
Liver, fresh, beef, fried, 4 oz.	114	260	29.8	12.0	6.0
Liverwurst, fresh, 4 oz.	114	350	18.4	29.0	2.0
Lobster, fresh, cooked in shell, 1 lb.	452	112	22.0	1.8	.4
fresh or canned, 4 oz.	114	106	21.0	1.7	.3

Food	Weight Gm.	Calories	Protein Gm.	Fat Gm.	Carbohydrate Gm.
Macaroni, cooked, 8-10 min., 1 cup	130	190	6.4	.6	39.0
cooked, 14-20 min., 1 cup	140	155	4.8	.6	32.0
Makeral, broiled w/butter, 4 oz.	114	266	24.6	17.8	0
Margarine, 1 tablespoon	14	100	.1	11.2	TR
Milk, cow's fresh, whole, 3.5% fat, 1 cup	246	158	8.5	8.5	11.8
whole, 3.7% butterfat, 1 cup	246	160	8.5	9.0	11.8
skim, 1 cup	246	88	8.8	.2	12.4
skim, half and half (2%), 1 cup	246	144	10.2	4.9	14.8
Milk, canned, condensed, sweetened, 1/2 cup	153	490	12.2	13.1	83.0
canned, condensed, unsweetened, 1 cup	126	172	8.8	9.8	12.2
Mushrooms, raw, sliced, 1 cup	68	19	1.8	.2	3.0
Mussels, raw, meat only, 4 oz.	114	107	16.2	2.5	3.8
Mustard, prepared, brown, 1 teaspoon	10	9	.6	.6	.5
prepared, yellow, 1 teaspoon	10	8	15	.4	.6
Noodles, egg, cooked, 1 cup	160	200	6.6	2.4	37.2
Oil, cooking, salad or veg., 1 tablespoon	14	124	0	14.0	0
Olives, canned or bottled, green, 2 oz.	57	65	.8	7.3	.8
Onions, mature, fresh, 1 average	110	40	1.6	.1	9.4
Orange juice, fresh, 6 oz. glass	186	86	1.3	.4	20.2
canned, sweetened, 6 oz. glass	186	97	1.3	.4	22.7
canned, unsweetened, 6 oz. glass	186	90	1.5	.4	20.7
frozen, unsweetened, 6 oz. glass	186	85	1.1	.4	20.0
Orange, grapefruit juice, canned, 6 oz. glass	185	94	.9	.2	22.4
frozen, unsweetened, diluted, 6 oz. glass	175	77	1.0	.2	18.3
Oranges, fresh, 1 average (2 4/5" diameter)	180	60	2.0	.2	16.0
Florida, 1 average (3" diameter)	210	75	1.5	.4	19.0
Oysters, canned, w/liquid, 4 oz.	114	87	9.7	2.5	5.6
Pancakes, from mix, 4" diameter cake:					
plain or buttermilk, prepared w/milk	45	90	2.7	2.5	14.4
plain or buttermilk, w/milk & egg	45	100	3.2	3.3	14.6
Peach nectar, canned, 6 oz. glass	185	89	.4	TR	22.9
Peaches, fresh, 1 average (2" diameter)	114	35	.7	.1	10.0
fresh, slices, 1 cup	177	67	1.1	.2	17.2
frozen, sweetened, slices, 8 oz.	227	200	9.1	.2	51.3
Peanut Butter, 1 tablespoon	14	82	3.5	7.1	2.6
Peanuts, roasted, shelled, 4 oz.	114	660	29.7	55.2	23.4
roasted, shelled, 1 cup	144	842	37.4	71.4	27.0
Pears, fresh, 1 average	182	100	1.2	.7	25.2
fresh, slices, 1 cup	164	100	1.1	.7	25.1
canned, in heavy syrup, slices, 1 cup	255	194	.5	.5	38.0
Peas, green, immature, raw, shelled, 1 cup	138	116	8.8	.7	19.9
fresh, boiled, drained, 1 cup	163	116	8.9	.8	19.7
dry, split, boiled, drained, 1 cup	194	223	15.5	.6	40.1
Pecans, shelled, 4 oz.	114	779	10.4	80.8	16.6
Peppers, hot, chili, green, raw, seeded, 4 oz.	114	42	1.5	.2	10.3
sweet, green, raw, 1 average	62	14	.7	.1	3.0
Perch, white, raw, meat only, 4 oz.	114	134	21.9	4.5	0
yellow, raw, meat only, 4 oz.	114	103	22.1	1.0	0
Pheasant, raw, meat only, 4 oz.	114	184	26.8	7.7	0
Pickle relish, sour, 1 tablespoon	15	3	.1	.1	.4
Pickle relish, sweet, 1 tablespoon	15	21	.1	.1	5.1
Pickles, cucumber, dill, 1 average (4" long)	133	15	.9	.3	2.9
Pies, frozen, baked, apple, 2 oz. slice	57	145	1.1	5.8	22.8
coconut custard, 2 oz. slice	57	142	3.4	6.8	16.8
Pineapple, raw, diced, 1 cup	140	73	.6	.3	19.2
canned, heavy syrup, crushed, 1 cup	262	194	.8	.3	50.8
frozen, sweetened, chunks, 1 cup	230	196	1.0	.2	51.0

Food	Weight Gm.	Calories	Protein Gm.	Fat Gm.	Carbohydrate Gm.
Pineapple juice, canned, unsweetened, 6 oz.	185	102	.7	.2	25.0
frozen, diluted, 6 oz.	175	81	.7	TR	22.4
Pineapple-orange juice drink, canned, 6 oz.	185	100	.4	.2	25.0
Pizza w/cheese, frozen, baked, 4 oz.	114	279	10.8	8.1	40.4
Plums, fresh, Damson, 1 average	60	36	3	.1	9.7
Popcorn, popped, plain, 1 cup	11	43	1.4	.6	8.4
popped, w/oil or butter, 1 cup	14	64	1.4	3.1	8.3
Pork, fresh, medium-fat class:					
chop, broiled, lean & fat, 4 oz. w/bone	114	297	18.6	23.6	0
chop, broiled, lean only, 4 oz. w/bone	114	148	16.8	8.4	0
roast, Boston butt, lean & fat, 4 oz.	114	403	25.7	32.6	0
Potato chips, 2 oz.	57	324	3.0	22.7	28.5
Potato sticks, 2 oz.	57	310	3.6	20.7	28.9
Potatoes, white, baked, w/skin, 1 small	100	93	2.6	.1	21.1
boiled, with skin, 1 small	100	75	2.0	.1	17.6
french-fried, 10 pieces	57	155	2.4	7.5	20.5
frozen, french-fried, heated, 17 pieces	85	187	3.0	7.1	28.6
frozen, hash browned, heated, 1 cup	200	448	4.0	23.0	58.0
Potatoes, sweet, baked, 1 average	110	155	2.3	.5	35.7
Pretzels, 2 oz.	57	222	5.6	2.6	43.3
Prune juice, canned or bottled, 6 oz.	192	148	.8	.2	36.5
Prunes, dehydrated, nugget-type, pitted, 4 oz.	114	390	3.8	.6	103.5
dried, w/pits, cooked, sweetened, 1 cup	258	444	2.1	.5	116.4
Pumpkin, fresh, pulp only, 4 oz.	114	30	1.1	.1	7.4
Radishes, fresh, 4 small	40	7	.4	TR	1.4
Pudding, starch base, chocolate w/milk, 1 cup	290	360	9.8	8.8	66.1
Raisins, natural, uncooked, 1 cup	143	413	3.6	.3	110.7
Raspberries, black, fresh, 1 cup	123	90	1.8	1.7	19.3
Rhubarb, raw, trimmed, 4 oz.	114	18	.7	.1	4.2
Rice, brown, cooked, 1 cup	168	200	4.2	1.0	42.8
white, long grain, cooked, 1 cup	169	179	3.5	.2	39.4
white, precooked, ready-to-serve, 1 cup	140	153	3.1	TR	33.9
Rolls, packaged, ready-to-serve, hard, 2 oz.	57	178	5.6	1.8	33.9
pan rolls, plain, 2 oz.	57	170	4.7	3.2	30.2
raisin, 2 oz.	57	157	3.9	1.6	32.1
sweet, 1 oz.	57	180	4.8	5.2	28.1
whole wheat, 2 oz.	57	146	5.7	1.6	29.8
Rolls, brown & serve, browned, 2 oz.	57	170	5.1	2.6	31.1
Salad dressing, bottled, French, 1 tablespoon	15	62	.1	5.8	2.6
Italian, 1 tablespoon	15	83	TR	9.0	1.0
mayonnaise, 1 tablespoon	15	108	.2	12.0	.3
Roquefort or blue cheese, 1 tablespoon	15	76	.7	7.8	1.1
Russian, 1 tablespoon	15	74	.2	7.6	1.6
thousand island, 1 tablespoon	15	75	.1	7.5	2.3
Salami, dry, 4 oz.	114	513	27.1	43.4	1.4
Salami, cooked, 4 oz.	114	354	19.9	29.2	1.6
Salmon, Atlantic, canned, w/liquid, 4 oz.	114	232	24.8	13.9	0
smoked, 4 oz.	114	200	24.6	10.6	0
Sardines, Atlantic, canned in oil, drained, 3 oz.	85	173	20.4	9.4	NA
Sauerkraut, canned, w/liquid, 4 oz.	114	20	1.1	.2	4.6
Sausage:					
brown-and-serve, browned, 4 oz.	114	481	18.8	43.1	3.2
country-styled, smoked, 4 oz.	114	393	17.2	35.4	0
Polish-style, 4 oz.	114	346	17.9	29.4	1.4
pork, links or bulk, cooked, 4 oz.	114	543	20.6	50.4	TR
Scallops, bay or sea, fresh, steamed, 4 oz.	114	128	26.4	1.6	NA

Food	Weight Gm.	Calories	Protein Gm.	Fat Gm.	Carbohydrate Gm.
Sesame seeds, dry, hulled, 4 oz.	114	660	20.7	60.6	20.0
Shad, canned, w/liquid, 4 oz.	114	172	19.2	10.0	0
Sherbert, orange, 1 cup	170	228	1.5	2.0	52.4
Shrimp, fresh, breaded, fried, 4 oz.	114	255	23.0	12.2	11.3
Soft drinks, carbonated, cola, 8 oz.	245	96	0	0	24.5
cream soda, 8 oz.	245	105	0	0	26.9
fruit flavored, 8 oz.	245	113	0	0	29.4
ginger ale & quinine water, 8 oz.	245	76	0	0	19.6
root beer, 8 oz.	245	100	0	00	25.7
Sole, raw, fillets, 4 oz.	114	89	18.9	.9	0
Soup, condensed, diluted, w/water or milk, 1 cup:					
bean w/pork, diluted w/water	249	167	8.0	5.7	21.7
beef broth, bouillon or consomme w/water	238	31	5.0	0	2.6
beef noodle, diluted w/water	238	67	3.8	2.6	6.9
chicken consomme, diluted w/water	238	21	3.3	TR	1.9
chicken, cream of, diluted, w/milk	238	174	7.1	10.0	14.0
chicken noodle, diluted w/water	238	62	3.3	1.9	7.9
chicken w/rice, diluted w/water	238	48	3.1	1.2	5.7
chicken, vegetable, diluted w/water	240	74	4.1	2.4	9.4
clam chowder, Manhatten, diluted w/water	240	79	2.2	2.4	12.0
clam chowder, New England, frozen, diluted w/milk	235	202	8.7	11.8	15.7
minestrone, diluted w/water	240	103	4.8	3.4	13.9
onion, diluted w/water	238	64	5.2	2.4	5.2
oyster stew, frozen, diluted w/milk	235	197	9.9	11.5	13.9
pea, green, diluted w/water	245	130	5.6	2.2	22.5
tomato, diluted w/water	240	86	1.9	2.4	15.4
vegetable beef, diluted w/water	240	77	5.0	2.2	9.4
Soy sauce, 1 tablespoon	14	9	.8	.2	1.2
Soybeans, young seeds, boiled, drained, 4 oz.	114	134	11.1	5.8	11.5
Spaghetti, cooked firm, 8-10 minutes, 1 cup	130	192	6.5	.7	39.1
cooked tender, 14-20 minutes, 1 cup	140	155	4.8	.6	32.2
canned in tomato sauce w/cheese, 8 oz.	227	172	5.0	1.4	34.9
Spinach, fresh, raw, chopped, 1 cup	52	14	1.7	.2	2.2
Squash, summer, fresh, white, cooked, mashed, 1 cup	238	38	1.7	.2	9.0
Strawberries, fresh, whole, capped, 1 cup	144	53	1.0	.7	12.1
frozen, sweetened, sliced, 8 oz.	227	247	1.2	.5	63.1
Sugar, brown, firm-packed, 1 cup	212	791	0	0	204.4
brown, firm-packed, 1 tablespoon	14	52	0	0	13.5
granulated, 1 cup	195	751	0	0	194.0
Sunflower seeds, hulled, 4 oz.	114	635	27.2	53.7	22.6
Syrups:					
cane, 1 tablespoon	20	53	0	0	13.6
maple, 1 tablespoon	20	50	0	0	13.0
table blend, chiefly corn syrup, 1 tablespoon	20	58	0	0	15.0
Tangerine juice, fresh, 6 oz.	186	80	.9	.4	18.8
Tangerine juice, frozen, sweetened, diluted, 6 oz.	170	78	.9	.3	18.4
Tangerines, fresh, whole, 1 average	114	39	.7	.2	9.7
Tartar sauce, 1 tablespoon	14	74	.2	8.1	.6
Tea, instant, 1 tablespoon dry	4	1	NA	TR	.4
Tomato juice, canned, 6 oz.	181	38	1.3	.2	9.1
Tomatoes, ripe, fresh, whole, 1 small	150	33	1.6	.3	7.0
Tuna fish, canned in oil, drained, 4 oz.	114	223	27.8	7.9	0
canned in water w/liquid, 4 oz.	114	144	31.8	.9	0
Turkey, fresh, dark meat only, roasted, 4 oz.	114	232	34.3	9.5	0
fresh, light meat only, roasted, 4 oz.	114	201	37.6	4.4	0
fresh, skin only, roasted, 2 oz.	57	256	9.6	23.8	0

Food	Weight Gm.	Calories	Protein Gm.	Fat Gm.	Carbohydrate Gm.
canned, boned, 4 oz.	114	231	23.9	14.3	0
potted, 4 oz.	114	283	9.9	21.9	0
pot pie, frozen, 8 oz. pie	227	447	13.2	23.6	45.6
Turnips, fresh, raw, slices, 1 cup	127	36	3.8	.4	6.4
Veal, fresh, flank, stewed, lean & fat, 4 oz.	114	446	27.2	36.9	0
Vegetable juice cocktail, canned, 6 oz.	181	31	1.6	.2	6.5
Waffles, frozen, 1 double waffle	50	127	3.6	3.1	21.0
Walnuts, black, shelled, 4 oz.	114	712	23.3	67.3	16.8
Watermelon, fresh, whole, 1 wedge	925	111	2.1	.8	27.2
Weakfish, broiled, meat only, 4 oz.	114	236	27.9	12.9	0
Yogurt, partially skim milk, 1 cup	249	125	8.5	4.2	12.9
Yogurt, whole milk, 1 cup	246	153	7.4	8.4	12.1

II
Fast Food Items — Kcal.

Item	Kcal.
Apple Turnover	286
Banana Split	560
Chicken	
Drumstick	224
Three piece	672
Dinner "with trimmings"	974
Snack	340
Cinnamon Roll	304
Donuts	240–270
Egg Sandwich	310
Fish	
and Chips	270
Filet	404
Sandwich	270
French Fries, small	212
Ham and Cheese	454
Hamburger	
Regular	250
Cheeseburger	307
Large-Super Large with Cheese	412–610
Hot Dog	290
Ice Cream	
Large Cone	360–394
Medium Cone	240–260
Small Cone, Most Flavors	160–220
Small Cone, Sherbet	134
One Dip, Most Flavors	146
One Dip, Sherbet	104
Milkshake	318
Roast Beef	
Regular Sandwich	424
Junior Sandwich	248
Large Sandwich	696
Taco, Specialities	
Taco	158
Enchirito	416
Frijoles	176
Turkey Sandwich	
Without Dressing	340
With Dressing	398

Note: The values provided above are approximations. When a range of values is provided and you are unsure of which number to select, determine and utilize the average of the two values.

III
Estimated Energy Expenditure for Selected Activities

Activity	I 90-109	II 110-129	III 130-149	IV 150-169	V 170-189	VI 190-209	VII 210+	Group Lbs.
Archery	3.2	3.7	4.2	4.7	5.3	5.9	6.5	
Badminton	4.8	5.3	6.2	7.1	7.9	8.7	9.5	
Baseball	3.5	3.8	4.4	5.0	5.6	6.1	6.6	
Basketball	6.5	7.7	8.9	10.1	11.3	12.5	13.6	
Bicycling 5.0 mph	3.2	3.6	4.1	4.6	5.1	5.6	6.2	
Bicycling 12.0 mph	6.8	8.0	9.2	10.4	11.6	12.8	14.0	
Bowling	4.2	5.1	6.1	7.1	8.0	9.0	10.2	
Boxing	9.0	10.7	12.2	13.9	15.6	17.0	18.8	
Calesthenics	4.2	5.1	6.0	6.9	7.8	8.7	9.6	
Canoeing Leisure	2.0	2.4	2.8	3.2	3.6	4.0	4.4	
Canoeing Intense	5.0	5.9	6.9	7.8	8.7	9.6	10.4	
Circuit Training	9.1	10.5	12.0	13.6	15.1	16.7	18.2	
Dance Social	5.0	5.8	6.7	7.6	8.5	9.4	10.3	
Dance Square	4.5	5.4	6.3	7.2	8.1	9.0	10.1	
Eating	1.1	1.3	1.5	1.7	1.9	2.1	2.3	
Fencing	5.2	6.5	7.8	9.1	10.4	11.7	14.4	
Field Hockey	6.4	7.8	8.8	10.0	11.2	12.4	14.0	
Fishing	2.9	3.4	3.9	4.5	5.0	5.5	6.2	
Football Moderate	3.0	3.9	4.8	5.7	6.6	7.5	8.8	
Football Intense	6.4	7.5	8.6	9.7	10.8	11.9	13.6	
Gardening	5.4	6.4	7.4	8.4	9.4	10.4	11.6	
Golf	4.1	4.8	5.5	6.2	6.9	7.7	8.4	
Gymnastics	3.1	3.7	4.3	4.9	5.5	6.1	7.3	
Handball	6.4	7.6	8.9	10.1	11.3	12.5	14.0	
Horseback Riding	5.3	6.2	7.2	8.1	9.0	10.0	11.1	
Judo/Karate	9.2	10.8	12.6	14.4	16.2	18.0	19.8	
Lying at Rest	1.1	1.3	1.5	1.7	1.9	2.1	2.3	
Mountain Climbing	6.4	7.7	9.0	10.3	11.6	12.8	14.2	
Music Playing Sitting	1.8	2.2	2.8	3.2	3.6	4.0	4.6	
Music Playing Standing	1.9	2.3	2.7	3.1	3.6	4.1	4.7	
Music Playing Drums	3.1	3.7	4.3	4.9	5.5	6.1	6.9	
Paddle Ball–Racquetball	6.4	7.8	9.2	10.6	12.0	13.4	16.6	
Painting	2.6	3.4	4.2	5.0	5.8	6.6	7.4	
Pool Billiards	1.3	1.6	1.8	2.1	2.4	2.6	3.2	
Rowing	6.4	8.4	10.5	12.5	14.5	16.6	18.8	
Running Cross Country	8.0	9.4	10.8	12.2	13.6	14.9	16.4	
Running 12 minute Mile	6.4	7.6	8.8	10.0	11.1	12.3	13.6	
Running 8 minute Mile	10.6	12.1	13.7	15.3	16.9	18.5	20.3	
Running 6 minute Mile	13.4	15.1	16.7	18.3	20.0	21.6	23.6	
Sailing	2.0	2.4	2.8	3.2	3.6	4.0	4.8	
Sitting Quietly	1.1	1.3	1.4	1.6	1.7	1.9	2.1	
Skating	5.2	5.6	7.0	8.4	9.8	11.2	14.6	
Skiing Downhill	6.8	7.8	8.8	9.8	10.8	11.8	14.2	
Skiing Cross Country	7.2	8.4	9.6	10.8	12.0	13.2	14.8	
Skin Diving	10.2	12.0	13.5	15.0	16.5	18.2	20.4	
Soccer	6.2	7.3	8.4	9.5	10.6	11.8	13.2	
Squash	9.4	11.3	13.2	15.1	17.1	19.0	21.4	
Standing Quietly	1.3	1.5	1.7	1.9	2.1	2.4	2.6	
Swimming Breast	7.8	9.2	10.6	11.0	13.4	14.8	16.4	
Swimming Crawl	7.2	8.3	9.4	10.5	11.6	12.7	14.2	
Swimming Tread	3.2	3.7	4.2	4.7	5.2	5.7	6.4	
Table Tennis	3.2	3.8	4.4	5.0	5.6	6.2	7.1	
Tennis	5.2	6.1	7.0	7.9	8.9	9.9	11.2	
Walking Slow	2.3	2.8	3.2	3.7	4.2	4.6	5.6	

Activity	I 90-109	II 110-129	III 130-149	IV 150-169	V 170-189	VI 190-209	VII 210+	Group Lbs.
Walking Medium	3.2	4.2	5.2	6.2	7.2	8.2	9.6	
Walking Fast	4.4	5.2	6.0	6.8	7.7	8.6	9.8	
Water Skiing	5.2	6.3	7.4	8.5	9.5	10.6	12.2	
Weight Training	5.0	6.1	7.2	8.2	9.3	10.4	12.0	
Wrestling	8.2	9.9	11.7	13.4	15.2	17.0	19.4	

Note: This chart provides an estimate of the number of calories burned per minute (energy expenditure) for various activities. The number of calories burned per minute is dependent upon several factors including metabolic type, body weight, and intensity of movement. The seven weight classifications above help provide a more valid estimate of the number of calories burned. In using this chart to develop an estimate of the total calories burned per day, expenditure values of similar activities can be substituted. Example: Substituting the values for sitting when determining caloric expenditure for similar activities such as knitting, sewing or typing.

EVALUATION SHEET
Personal Appraisal No. 14

Name _____

Date _____

Lifetime Participation

  I. *Title:* Caloric Balance

  II. *Objectives:*

  III. *Results:*

    Total Kcal consumed for five days   _____

    Average Kcal consumed per day   _____

    Total Kcal burned for five days   _____

    Average Kcal burned per day   _____

    SUMMARY:

    Average calories injested per day   _____

    Average calories burned per day   _____

                                                      _____ Difference

    Check one: Excess in calories   _____

                 Deficit in calories   _____

IV. *Analysis:*

    1. Do you find significance in the result of this personal appraisal? Explain.

    2. Have you recently gained weight? Yes _____ (Lbs _____) No _____
       Describe the reasons for your weight gain.

    3. Have you recently lost weight? Yes _____ (Lbs _____) No _____
       Describe the cause of your weight loss.

    4. Have you maintained your present body weight for a substantial length of time? Yes _____ (Years _____ Months _____) No _____

       a. If yes, is your present body weight ideal? Lbs. _____
          Explain!

V. *Implications:*

    1. If you do not presently maintain your ideal body weight, what stimulus would be necessary for you to start either a weight gain or weight reduction program?

    2. List the dietary habit and pattern changes you can employ, which will help you to control your body weight.

10
EMOTIONAL AND PSYCHOLOGICAL VALUES

For many years, educators have embraced the concept of the "whole person." This theory is founded upon the precept that the mind and body function as a unit. Physical health occurs to an extent as a result of physical activity, but does activity influence our state of mental health? We know that many health problems are psychosomatic in nature. Problems such as ulcers, headaches, gastric upsets, are functional since specific physical causes cannot be identified. State of mind, ability to adapt to stress, feelings of self—have a great influence on one's physical health. The whole man theory implies that physical activity can influence our mental and emotional wellbeing. Evidence is constantly acccumulating, which supports this theory.

Each of us is born with an innate drive toward activity. The infant first learns through movement. There is a need to move, to be active. Physical and mental growth is stimulated through movement. As the infant develops, movement forms illicit pleasant sensations, feelings of success, and positive responses from parents.

The young child develops the feeling of fatigue after he has been vigorously active. Adults often exhibit the sensation of fatigue before activity. What happens during the transition from youth to adulthood which permits this contradiction to occur? Could it be the feeling of tiredness that often results without physical cause is based on psychological reasons? We are tired at times because we want to be tired. What has happened to the innate drive towards activity?

Most adults will not indulge in activity unless it has personal meaning and value. Social benefits, which result from personal associations and friendships, are realized through participation in sport activities and competition. Habits and attitudes developed through social interaction readily transfer to real life situations. This potential for social development and its effect on mental health, seems to be positive and may assist us to deal more effectively and compassionately with our family and peers.

A sense of well-being and euphoria is often experienced at the conclusion of physical activity. This pleasant feeling seems to be closely related to emotional changes. These changes are characterized by alterations in mood states which may appear periodically or with regularity. They may modify considerable areas of personality which vary in duration and intensity. However, conclusive evidence does not show that these mood modifications will develop favorable personality traits. This area of investigation is based solely upon short term studies leaving an area in which a great deal of research is needed.

STRESS ADAPTATION

Stress is a condition in which a number of hormonal reactions occur in assisting our body to adapt to changes in our physical and emotional environment. These hormonal reactions help us to confront, withstand and adjust to changing circumstances and conditions (stressors) which occur daily throughout life. These "stressors" trigger the bodies adaptive responses. Stress resulting from pleasant or stimulating experiences are termed EUSTRESS and are usually not destructive. DISTRESS is the opposite of EUSTRESS and can be extremely unpleasant and harmful.

The bodies adaptive mechanisms are not finite. When stress occurs, wounds are inflicted and internal scars remain. As the intensity and duration of stress increases, the more devastating its effects. Our bodies can be compared to a chain in that when increasing stress is applied, the weakest link will break first. In a manner owing to heredity or environment, our weakest organ or system is the most likely to break down when confronted with excessive biological stress. For this reason, individuals develop different states from identical stressors. In some, the heart may be affected while in others, the gastrointestinal tract or nervous system may experience disease. Chronic and intense stress may result in heart attack, hypertension, peptic ulcer, mental breakdown and even cancer.

Signs of Distress

The following list demonstrates the wide variety of signs that may be experienced by individuals exposed to high levels of stress. These signs are generally due to the malfunction of the most vulnerable organs and systems of our body. When these signs become chronic or multiple signs are experienced, the human body is in danger of serious disorders.

1. increased use of prescription drugs (tranquilizers, amphetamines)
2. increased use of alcohol
3. increased smoking
4. insomnia
5. migrane headaches
6. frequent urination
7. increase or decrease in appetite
8. nervous ticks
9. trembling
10. pain in lower back or neck
11. impotence
12. decrease in sex drive
13. impulsive behavior
14. irritability
15. lack of concentration
16. accident proneness
17. excessive fatigue
18. stress induced speech problems (stuttering)

Physical activity develops our ability to adapt to stress and provides a means of emotional release. It can act as an escape valve or a chance to momentarily change our area of concentration. There are times when each of us is in need of release from a frustrating situation or a vexing problem. An extremely effective method of gaining relief is through participation in physical activity. Using physical activity as a diversion may not solve the problem, however, it does provide the opportunity for psychological rejuvenation. While vigorous activity influences physical condition, it may also assist one in maintaining a clarity of mind and purpose. When again confronting the original problem, the approach to a solution for the dilemma may be more objective and the problem may not seem as intense as it once appeared.

It has been demonstrated that one's ability to adapt to stress is developed through involvement in physical activity. In our tremendously complex and rapidly changing world, everyday living can be shown to be a constant cycle of pleasures and tensions. Pleasure may be the result of success, of positive personal relationships, of the lack of friction and problems that produce frustration. Pressures of tension and stress result from a variety of sources. Our environment is filled with complexity involving crowded city living, rapidly changing social mores, confusing dilemmas of law and a very slowly responding government. Our lives revolve around emotional interaction characterized by love, hate and fear, as well as other emotions reflected in behavior.

Stress is also produced through participation in sports and physical activity. Stress ranges from the psychological tension of the distance runner in tolerating fatigue, to the pressure a basketball player experiences when called upon to convert a foul shot in order to win in the last seconds of a game. Although physical activity causes stress, participation in regular exercise conditions the stress adaptation mechanism which acts to ease or diffuse the stress of daily living. Conversely, a lack of physical activity may result in less ability to withstand stress. Research encourages us to conclude that the process of stress adaptation initiated through active living may result in the improvement of emotional health.

Social Implication

Indulging in physical exercise has great value in a social context. It can aid in our ability to interact with others, thereby helping to satisfy basic emotional needs, and creating more accessible pathways for communication and understanding. Physical activity has the potential for being a positive force in personality development and provides the opportunity for spontaneous emotional expression. Many studies have shown a relationship between personal-social characteristics and physical-motor traits for college age students. Generally, this research indicated that students high on physical-motor tests tended to be extroverted, sociable, dependable, tolerant, active, and competitive; they were prone to be leaders and popular with their peers.

We feel strongly that there is an improvement of psychological states by means of exercise programs. Through active living, we can provide an atmosphere in which our emotions and state of psychological well-being will thrive and assist us in contributing to humanity.

Selected References

Hanks, M., and Eckland, B. Athletics and social participation in the educational attainment process. *Sociology of Education,* 1976, 49, 271–294.

Kroll, W. The stress of high performance athletics. In P. Klovora and J. V. Daniel (Eds.) Coach, athlete, and the sport psychologist. Champaign: Human Kinetics Publishers, 1979.

Maccoby, E., T. Jacklin, C. N. The psychology of sex differences. Stanford, Calif.: Stanford Press, 1974.

Scott, J. Men and women in sport: The manhood myth. In G. H. McGlynn (Ed.), *Issues in Physical Education and Sport,* Palo Alto, Calif.: National Press Book, 1974.

Sonstroem, R. J. The validity of self-perceptions regarding physical and athletic ability. *Medicine and Science in Sports,* 1978, 10, 197–102

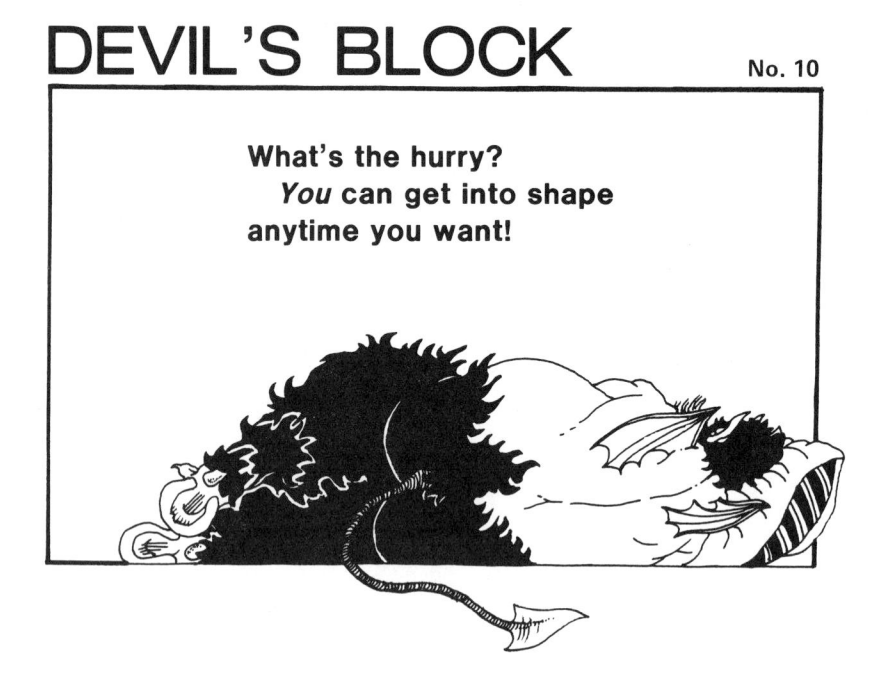

DEVIL'S BLOCK No. 10

What's the hurry?
***You* can get into shape anytime you want!**

11
CHEMICAL INFLUENCES AND CONDITIONING

We have recently witnessed the proliferation of information in which the use and abuse of chemicals have been debated. A vast number of articles have been published in which the controversial nature of this subject has been highlighted. Divergent views still persist, however the accumulation of research is providing us with valid and reliable data for which a common base of agreement now exists. The body of knowledge, which is now being compiled, consists of many proven facts and concepts which may be translated into healthful behavior. If this body of knowledge were reflected in our daily behavior, our society would realize much less trauma, and experience a decline in social ills.

We use the term chemicals to describe all substances which enter the circulatory system of the human organism. Chemical intake can be oral, inhaled through the nose, enter via injection or through a break in the skin. The effect of these substances vary in type, duration and intensity. Within the context of conditioning and athletic performance, these substances include medicines, alcohol, drugs and narcotics, nicotine, vitamins, minerals, and some foods. Some chemicals can be utilized in a positive manner such as aspirin in relieving pain. Virtually all chemicals can be abused incurring detrimental effects to the body. The results of chemical use range from maintaining life to adverse side effects, including death as in the case of barbituates and heroin.

We are often unaware of the consequences that may occur with chemical abuse. This is vividly substantiated when we note the many years it took before the effects of smoking on the lungs and circulatory system were proven. Morphine was used as a pain reliever for a long time before its addictive potential was realized. The risk of using the pill as a method of contraception has only recently been demonstrated. At times, we delude ourselves into believing we are immune to the detrimental effects of chemical use. We tell ourselves while others may suffer, it can't happen to us! This logic is self-defeating.

Research has demonstrated that many chemical substances have a greater potential of causing physical and mental harm than their use warrants for wholesome or health-related benefits. When this is the case, or potentially beneficial chemicals are abused, the negative effects elicit a decline in conditioning levels and a related decrease in total health. Chemical use can be considered antagonistic to positive health when unwanted side effects are greater than potential benefits.

Our society, with its great emphasis on competitive sports, has inspired some individuals to explore ways of increasing physical output. Although some of the measures used to increase performance and capacity are reprehensible to many of us, others which have been administered foster human improvement and are in the best interest of the individual. These **ergogenic** aids can be foodstuffs, substances, or methods of approach which result or are purported to result in increased work output. Ergogenic aids function in one of two ways; by reducing inhibitory forces that restrict performance and by increasing work capacity of the muscles.

Human beings are notorious in searching for the "golden alexir," the "short cut to perfection," the "gimmick" or that "something extra." Athletes have experimented with ergogenic aids for hundreds of years. The first recorded death from drug usage in athletics occurred in the late 1890's when a cyclist in Britian died as a result of using the stimulant ephedrine. Other tragedies involving the use of drugs in athletics have since occurred while thousands of less serious health problems have also resulted. Drug related health problems have included accidents, organ and tissue destruction and impairment, addiction, hindered performance, and unwanted side effects.

It is difficult to identify research that demonstrates safe athletic improvement as a result of drug usage. One certainty has been proven, losers rely on drugs much more than do winners.

International Sport Federations frown on drug use in athletic programs. The British have stated that the use of any chemical substance not normally present in the body can be categorized as "doping" and has no place in the world of sport.

Certainly all of us would appreciate any easy route to improved conditioning and motor performance, however there is no better road to improved health than through proper nutrition and persistent training. In a liberal sense, adequate rest, proper nutrition and excellent training programs can genuinely be labeled ergogenic.

It is not our intention to consider training methods as aids, but rather to discuss the influence of chemicals upon performance and conditioning. We have listed below examples of chemical substances used by some individuals involved with conditioning and sports. Due to the lack of controlled research in a number of these areas, some of our views have been derived from empirical evidence.

1. *Amphetamines*—These drugs function as a central nervous system stimulant in reducing fatigue and increasing capacity for performing work. The evidence of improvements of strength, fatigue inhibition, coordination and improved performance is at best contradictory. In light of the above, and the dangers of addiction, diminishing overstrain warning, and possible collapse, using amphetamines as an ergogenic aid seems inadvisable.

2. *Alcohol*—Alcohol is the most abused drug in this country. This results from its widespread acceptance which unfortunately has caused many authorities to retreat from public pronouncement of alcohols toxicity and its impact on society. In terms of athletics and sport, the use of alcohol is generally not recommended, however some sportsmen have described positive effects from drinking beer after workouts or during long endurance events. Although the ergogenic benefits of beer lack substantiation of research, we do know that there is real danger of tolerance increase. In addition, the concept of alcohol use in athletics incur the threat of breakdowns in training and performance.

3. *Anabolic Steroids*—Some of these substances have the ability of producing androgenic or masculine characteristics and an anabolic or protein building potential. Synthetic steroids have been produced in which androgenic effects have decreased while anabolic effects have increased. Today, many of these synthetic steroids, which purportedly produce increased muscular mass and strength are in vogue with some of our champion athletes. The ergogenic effects of these steroids have not received conclusive scientific support. While the results of steroid use are contradictory, the potentially severe side effects add a dangerous risk factor.

4. *Caffeine*—Caffeine is used as a diuretic and central nervous system stimulant in medicine. It has been demonstrated that this drug adversely effects motor coordination and cardio-respiratory function.

5. *Vitamins and Minerals*—It seems obvious that any negative effects on conditioning and performance, resulting from vitamin and mineral deficiencies, would be eliminated through proper diet or vitamin supplements. The value of excess vitamin intake in improving conditioning and performance remains unsubstantiated.

6. *Wheat Germ Oil*—There are those who have attributed wonderful benefits to diets supplemented with wheat germ, soybean and corn oil. Although these substances may aid a deficient diet, there is little evidence to support their use as supplements.

7. *Sugar Feeding*—Sugar helps furnish the fuel used by muscles while performing work. It has been demonstrated that sugar will add to performance in activities requiring endurance. During long continuous activities, a slight break whereby one would ingest strongly sweetened tea with lemon, will provide energy thereby increasing performance.

8. *Water*—Performance in physical activities which require vigorous endurance exercise causes water loss through perspiration. This allows for a rapid onset of fatigue and exhaustion. Contrary to some training practices, drinking water during vigorous exercise can be beneficial.

9. *Salt*—Lowered levels of salts in the body causes a decrease in energy output, indicating that the ingestion of salt may be a wise precaution.

10. *Cigarette Smoking*—The adverse effects of smoking on conditioning and performance have been purported for many years. Research confirms many of these concerns. Moderate to heavy smoking over a period of time has been shown to result in the following:

   a. Reduction in the oxygen-carrying capacity of the lungs
   b. Decreased total lung and breathing capacity
   c. Increased heart rate
   d. Increased systolic and diastolic blood pressure
   e. Decreased endurance performance
   f. Decreased response to training

11. *Smoking Marijuana*—Research has provided us with massive evidence that marijuana is not the harmless transgression that many believe it to be. Our nation has become the most pervasive drug-abusing society in history and marijuana is the most abused drug. Users almost never realize its detrimental effects and for some the most serious side effects may not appear for many years. Marijuana produces a variety of symptoms which manifest themselves differently among individuals. The type and severity of side effects are dependent upon potency, frequency of smoking and length of time of indulgence. The frequency and length of time are of extreme importance since the cannabinoids in marijuana are fat soluable and tend to remain in the body. It takes up to 30 days for the body to completely dispose of the THC (active chemical in marijuana) from one joint. This means that habitual smokers build up tremendous amounts of cannabinoids in the cells. They tend to accumulate in cell membranes which are 60% fat and inhibit the entrance of proteins. Research indicated that marijuana may promote serious physical and psychological effects. It has been shown to cause genetic mutation and impair lung, brain and reproductive function. Ironically, users scoff at the research and the most ominous note is that great numbers of our youth are unconcerned when faced with possible deterioration of their body. Little research has been completed to date which provides valid information concerning the effects of marijuana on physical performance. Marijuana use results in an increased heart rate. Heavy use may result in increased systolic and diastolic blood pressure. Studies have shown that a drop in physical work capacity resulting from smoking marijuana may be explained by the changes in heart rate and blood pressure.

12. *Oxygen*—The advantage of administering oxygen before and during recovery has not been supported in available research. Evidence has demonstrated that improved performance can result from breathing pure oxygen during participation, however, this seems impractical in its administration.

In Chapter Two we have considered the concept of ecology and the preservation of one of our greatest natural resources; our health and productivity. The misuse of some ergogenic substances constitute the pollution of our bodies and a corresponding reduction in our potential for personal and societal improvement and growth.

While we recognize that chemicals have great value in relieving suffering and combating disease, we recommend as a general rule the maintenance of the body in its natural state. The human body thrives on use, replenishes itself but should not be abused. Until research demonstrates conclusively and without contradiction that chemical substances can improve conditioning and performance, with no risk of unwanted side effects, their use should be discouraged.

A wonderous and overwhelming feeling of satisfaction can be experienced when our accomplishments approach the heights of our potential without the assistance of external and artificial aids. When reflecting on these thoughts, it becomes easy to find agreement in the statment, "Let's get high on activity."

Selected References

Bowers, R., Reardon, J. Effects of methadrostenolone (dianobol) on strength development and aerobic capacity. (Abstract of paper presented at the 19th annual meeting of American College of Sports Medicine). *Medicine and Science in Sport.,* 4:54, 1972.

Cooper, G. R. and Mowbray, K. W. Effects of iron *supplementation* and activity on serum iron depletion and hemoglobin levels in female athletes. *Research Quarterly,* 1978, 49, 114–118.

Morgan, W. P. (Ed.) Ergogenic aids and muscular performance. New York: Academic Press, 1972.

O'Shea, J. Anabolic steroid: Effects of competitive swimmers. Nutrition Reports International. 1 (6): 337–342, 1970.

Stromme, S. B.; Meen, H. D., and Aakvaqq, A., Effects of androgenic—anabolic steroid on strength and development and plasma testosterone levels in normal males. *Medicine and Science in Sport.* 6(3): 203–208, 1974.

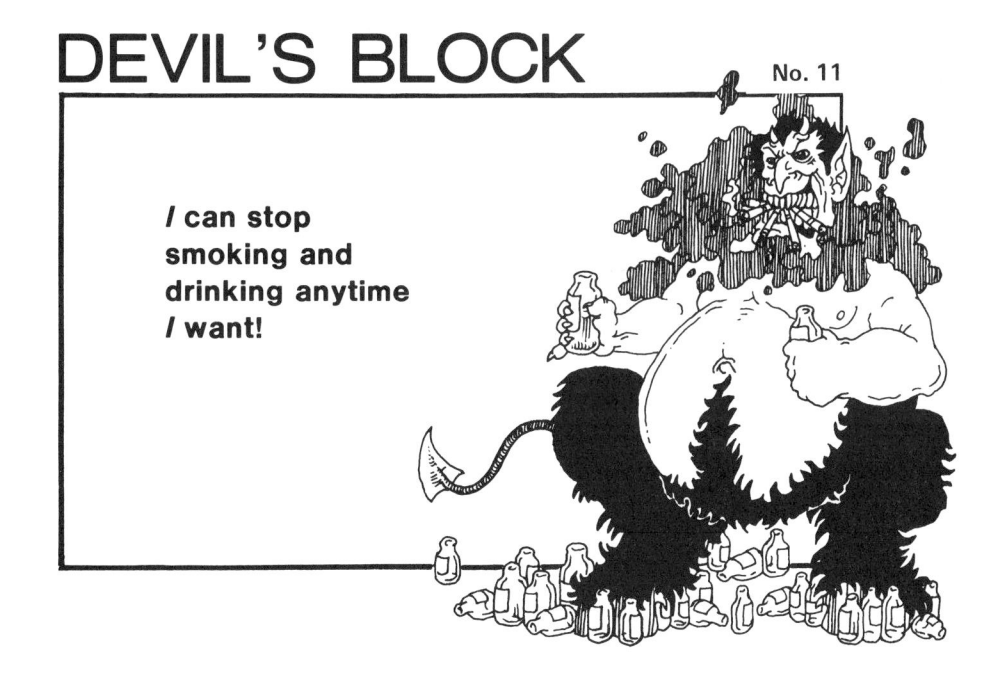

DEVIL'S BLOCK   No. 11

I can stop smoking and drinking anytime I want!

PROFILE CHART

Profile of Individual's Results in the Thirteen Self-Appraisal Tests

Personal Appraisals	Attitude	Body Image	Cardio-Respiratory (12-Min. Run)	Cardio-Respiratory (Recovery Rate)	Flexibility	Muscular Strength	Muscular Endurance I	Muscular Endurance II	Speed	Coordination	Agility	Balance	Explosive Power	Posture	Weight Control	Comments
	I	II	III$_A$	III$_C$	IV$_A$	V	VI$_I$	VI$_{II}$	VII	VIII	IX	X	XI	XII	XIII	
270		1	1	1	1	1	1	1	1	5	1	5	1	1	3	Range of Excellence
243														2		
216		2	2	2	2	2	2	2	2		2		2	4		
189		2	3	2	3	3	3	3		4	3	4	3	3		
134	3	4	3		3	4	3	4	4	3	3	3	4	4	5-6	Mean
108					4		4				4			5		
81		5	4		5	5	5	5	2	2	5				7-8	
54	4	6	5	6	5	6	6	5	1	5	6	7	6	9		Range of Deep Concern
	5		5		6		6			1						

Plot on the graph your score on each of the personal appraisals.

True understanding is: "when we see ourselves not as what we are—but as what we can eventually become."

SECTION II—CORE CONDITIONING PROGRAM
PUTTING YOURSELF TOGETHER

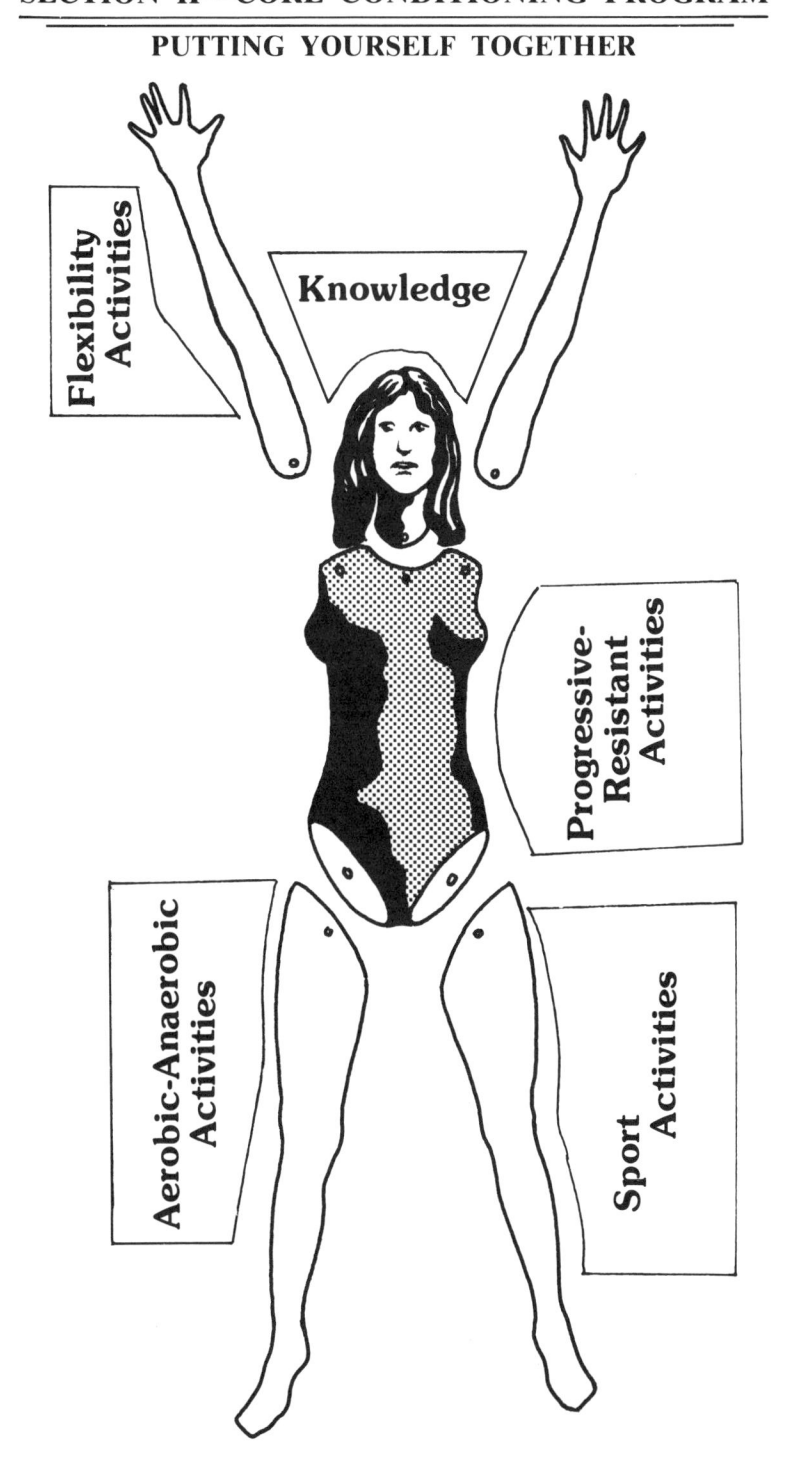

Knowledge

Flexibility Activities

Progressive-Resistant Activities

Aerobic-Anaerobic Activities

Sport Activities

Section II
CORE CONDITIONING PROGRAM

Few of us have designed lifetime activity programs through which we endeavor to increase or maintain high levels of condition. This is unfortunate since these programs may require little time, can be extremely enjoyable and most importantly, provide a multitude of health related benefits.

The intent of Section II is to introduce our readers to activities designed to provide a foundation upon which all principles of performance and physical conditioning are derived. We feel strongly that you should incorporate in your lifestyle the following three program areas and remain involved in some form of the same activities throughout life. These experiences are designed, not only as a basis for achieving a high level of conditioning, but also for the improvement of performance skills.

Program Experience I—II—III

"The Golden Triangle"

```
                    I  Static Stretching
                   /\
                  /  \
                 / ↑  \
                /      \
               / Flexibility \
              /          \
             /            \
            / Cardio-Respiratory \
           /   Efficiency    \
  Aerobic-/  Muscular Strength and  \ Progressive
 Anaerobic/II    Endurance ——→ III \ Resistance
         /_____\
```

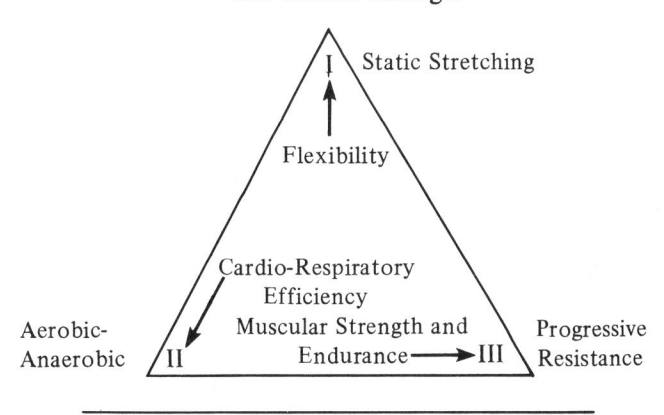

We refer to these three training arenas as the "Golden Triangle" since gold strongly infers the concept of richness or wealth. Continuous involvement in some form of the "Core Program" can help provide each of us with a wealth of quality experiences throughout our lives.

PREVENTIVE MAINTENANCE

THROUGH THE "GOLDEN TRIANGLE"

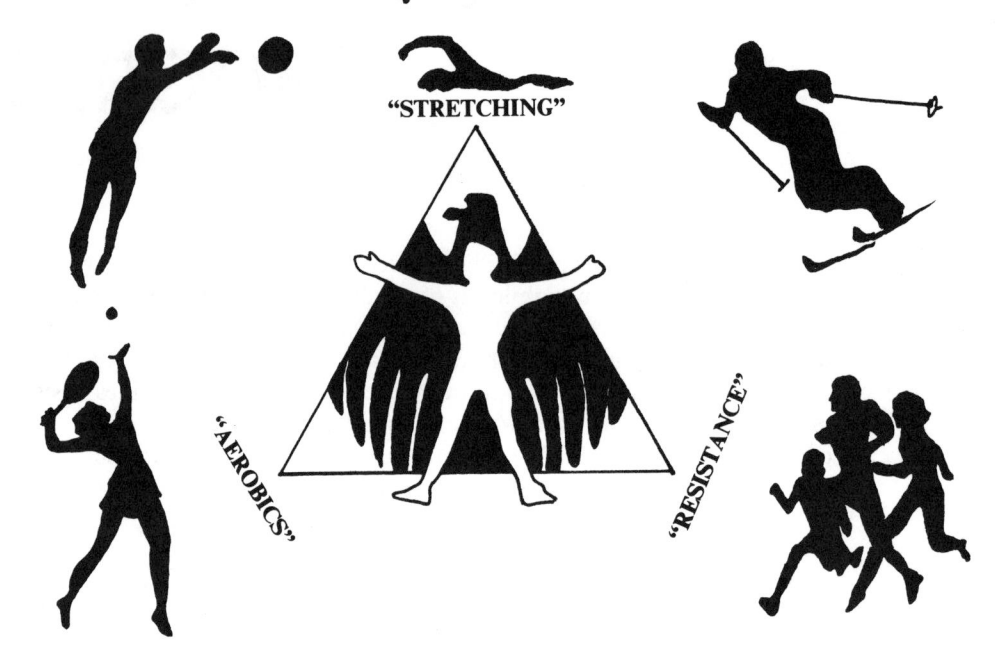

"STRETCHING"

"AEROBICS"

"RESISTANCE"

PUT THE "ODDS" IN YOUR FAVOR

PREVENT INJURY | DELAY FATIQUE | ENHANCE PERFORMANCE | RESIST DISEASE | ASSIST CONVALESENCE

12
PREVENTIVE MAINTENANCE

CONCEPT OF PREVENTIVE (MEDICINE) MAINTENANCE

Participation in the program areas of the "Golden Triangle" can be interpreted as "preventive (medicine) maintenance" which is fast becoming the key to a lifetime of positive health and vitality.

Modern science and medical knowledge have given all of us a taste of the perennial dream, the prolongation of life. The critical question may not be whether we can simply prolong our lives in order to reach advanced age, but rather the quality of life we will experience as we progress in years. Will we have sufficient energy? Will we be agile? Will our skeletal structure withstand constant pressure? Will we harbor degenerative heart disease? Will we be crippled by muscle spasms and arthritic agonies? Will we be susceptible to constant injury? Will we experience regression in our mental faculties?—or Will we be fortunate and remain alert, flexible, vigorous and find satisfaction and pleasure in living? The key to overcoming what many sometimes accept as the symptoms of age, is to keep the body functioning at its maximal potential as long as it remains alive. In working towards this goal, emphasis should be focused on preventive measures. Millions of dollars are spent annually in the pursuit of research to determine cause and cure. While these areas are highly important, logic dictates that more effort and resources be allocated for preventive maintenance.

The Epidemic Syndrome

If an epidemic were suddenly to strike this country killing thousands, permanently disabling millions, and incapacitating many others, it would be immediately recognized as a serious threat to our national economy and social structure. A state of emergency would be declared, and the nation as a whole would mobilize in an all out effort to combat the problem. In spite of great efforts to make individuals aware of the necessity of taking action to improve health and fitness, the general public still tends to remain apathetic. Poor health and lack of fitness with resultant illness and injury take a toll in human resources equivalent if not greater than the ravages of the hypothetical epidemic.

Unlike epidemics, which are usually concentrated in one area, poor health, and lack of fitness prevails throughout the country. Unlike either a war or a plague, which are highly visible and instant in effect, poor health and lack of fitness cannot be attributed to a single dramatic cause that suddenly disrupts normal conditions. They are incidious working like a slowly developing cancer with deleterious effects upon our society. The belief that ill health and poor fitness happens to the other person seems to prevail. Since these conditions are not contagious, it is easy to feel that with minimal effort and care we will be lucky enough to avoid the eventual problems which can result. For these reasons, most individuals remain more or less indifferent to this country's consistently high incident of poor health/fitness. In reality, these conditions should be a matter of grave concern to all citizens and we should all be stimulated to preventive action.

Preventing Pitfalls of Participation

Although one may be eager to participate in sports, individuals are often impatient with the conditioning exercises and practice sessions necessary to develop the strength, flexibility, cardio-respiratory capacity and skill required for preventive measures on the playing field.

Individuals should be cautioned not to engage in any sport activity until they have made every possible effort to ensure they are adequately conditioned as well as sufficiently skilled. (You get in shape to play a sport, you do not play the sport to get in shape). Many people experience difficulty while participating because they fail to realize that lack of conditioning and skill in sports demands unnecessary effort. This causes extraneous movement and awkwardness which may lead to a rapid onset of fatigue and increased vulnerability to injury.

Acquiring minimal skills can often lead to a dangerous complacency. For example, the person who manages to pass a 50 yard swimming test develops unjustifiable faith in his proficiency and may begin to take foolhardy chances. Because he fares well in supervised swimming areas, he erroneously assumes that he has enough skill to risk swimming in unguarded waters. Individuals must learn to accept their limitations and to recognize the chance of overexerting themselves and attempting feats beyond their ability. With proper knowledge, they can understand that the effort required to improve conditioning will be greatly rewarded, not only by a greater awareness of personal safety, but by the increased enjoyment that comes from doing things well.

Preventive Maintenance Through the "Golden Triangle"

The programs of the "Golden Triangle" are the prerequisites for preventive maintenance. Good health practices must go hand in hand with the program experiences of the "Golden Triangle." Adequate rest, a well-balanced diet, abstinence from nicotine, alcohol and other harmful substances, are an integral part of the conditioning process. The concept of the "Golden Triangle" as preventive maintenance can be exemplified in the following principles:

1. Developing good health and total fitness put the odds in your favor for living a better life.
2. To provide greater recuperative powers during the convalescent period if and when illness or injury occur.
3. To be better able to cope emotionally, when illness or injury occur.
4. To increase flexibility which will aid in resisting injury which often results from extreme movements of body segments.
5. Increased cardio-respiratory capacity will aid in resisting fatigue and the onset of degenerative disease.
6. Adequate muscular strength and endurance will help prevent undue fatigue and undue soreness and strain. Fatigue is a factor which leaves one more vulnerable to illness and injury.

7. To be able to recognize ones own strengths and limitations which hopefully will provide the "common sense" needed to know how far to extend oneself in any activity.
8. Exercise from cradle to grave, should serve as a vicarious outlet for tensions and can be thought of as the simplest "preventive measure."
9. "You get in shape to play a sport (i.e., tennis), you do not play the sport to get in shape." If the participant would recognize and adhere to this principle, great strides would be made to reduce the incidence of injury and to make participation a more pleasurable experience.

Focus and Insights

We have selected the "Golden Triangle" of activities as the Core Program with the intent of having each person experience joy, well-being and a sense of self-confidence. Such a program, we trust will develop and acquire a positive attitude toward remaining physically active, while at the same time, reaching for a high level of conditioning. A deep feeling of satisfaction and accomplishment occurs as we reach higher levels of physical capabilities and conditioning. To produce "high levels of conditioning," certain principles must be understood.

Principle 1—Acceptance of a starting point: Each of us should recognize our starting point. We cannot live in the past or attempt to immediately regain the levels of physical accomplishments we once knew. We must admit to the reality of our present state, and through a carefully planned progressive program of activity, build upon this. For example:

1. The outstanding athlete, when confronted by an accident, injury or illness, cannot reflect back to past glories. They must determine their new starting point (the limitations they are now under)—and through selected activities, improve the qualities so vital to happiness.
2. The elder statesmen should not sit and merely reflect upon how at twenty years of age they were able to run, jump and play. They should carefully analyze their present condition and then rededicate themselves to a more fulfilling life.
3. Students and young adults, while appreciating the efforts of the accomplished athlete, should not allow this to serve as a deterrent to their individual improvement. "I can never be as good as that—so therefore, why try," or "She's a natural, so therefore I could never gain that level of achievement."

Each individual should realize the following: "I am an individual, unique in many ways, I have strengths, and I have weaknesses, I have certain limitations, but also great potential. I can accept myself as I am today, but through living actively, I will improve the qualities of my life."

In this context you judge accomplishment, not upon the performance of others, but from the improvement you have made.

Principle 2—Reaction to physical discomfort: As we initiate new activities, we will experience muscular soreness, "aches and pains" creating discomfort. With experience one will be able to distinguish between this discomfort, opposed to symptoms of injury or illness. The aches, pains, and soreness resulting from physical activity, is the body's way of indicating that we are now exposing muscles to different patterns, and indicates how relatively inactive we have been. Soreness of this nature is rapidly eliminated as we persist in the training program. Sadly, the route taken by many is to "lie down until the feeling goes away."

Principle 3—Breaking the exercise barrier: As we initiate activity programs, we will be confronted by difficulties. We may start with a great deal of vigor and enthusiasm, however in a short period of time a vital decision must be made! We may experience soreness, we may become tired, we may even feel the program is far beyond our capabilities. We may reach the point of asking ourselves, "is it worth it?" Before vigorous physical activity can become a pleasurable experience, we must break through this "exercise barrier." This is the stage in which some of us decide to curtail participation. This is a serious mistake in judgment resulting in adverse effects and making resumption of activity more difficult.

To break through and overcome the "exercise barrier," to push beyond, makes training a valued experience rather than a chore. Naturally, we would like to eliminate as much discomfort as possible. The following measures should limit the incidence of discomfort to a minimum:

1. Progression in activity is important. Add length and intensity as tolerance is established.
2. We all have varying degrees of ability to tolerate pain. Many agree that those who have achieved the highest pinnacle of success in athletics have a high "threshold of pain." The lower our "threshold of pain," the more careful we should be in the progression and intensity of our workouts.
3. The choice is yours! Some discomfort is a natural phenomenon as we become actively involved. The better our state of fitness, the less discomfort we will experience and the time interval for the removal of any aches or soreness will be shortened.

Delayed Discomfort

Perseverance is perhaps the key concept in the maintenance and development of fitness and conditioning. The ability to continue in vigorous activity programs with regularity is difficult for many people. Simply continuing fitness programs, long enough to break through the exercise barrier, seems impossible for many. Others, frightened by the thought of exercise due to negative experiences in sport activities or physical education class, reject the prospect of initiating a program even though they accept the concept of improved health through vigorous activity. For some, exercise is time consuming, boring, fatiguing, difficult, and even painful. This need not be the case. Individuals do not have to expose themselves to negative experiences in the pursuit of health and fitness.

Delayed discomfort is an approach to entering into exercise programs in a manner designed to lessen or eliminate physiological and psychological discomfort. This approach encourages individuals to use common sense, set realistic goals, progress slowly but steadily, chart progress and generally ease into an active lifestyle with a minimum of discomfort and a maximum of enjoyment. The key to delayed discomfort is to cease activity when discomfort occurs. For some, activity would end with the onset of perceptions of fatigue or soreness. Others with a high threshold of pain might desire to continue activity until intense levels of discomfort occur. However, the untrained and deconditioned person should reduce or cease exercise as soon as feelings of discomfort cause them to no longer enjoy the activity.

This approach to fitness becomes highly successful when care is taken to measure and record achievement. The distance traveled, length of time or number of repetitions accomplished before the onset of discomfort for each area of exercise is charted. As the body begins to make physiological changes (training effects) and the ability to tolerate stress is increased, perceptions of discomfort are delayed as one becomes able to increase the duration or intensity of exercise. With precise record keeping, individuals will note improvement and begin to recognize the onset of the conditioning process.

Utilizing this unique approach, perceptions of discomfort can be reduced or eliminated so that individuals are able to participate for longer periods without having to subject themselves to pain, exhaustion and stress. We have, in effect, eliminated a major portion of the training barrier; physical and psychological discomfort.

Core Programs

The activities composing the "Golden Triangle" should be a requirement for all! The term requirement may elicit a negative reaction. It may be interpreted by some to negate a true concern for individual differences. This is far from true, for we have a deep concern for the individual. To function effectively the body needs physical activity. This need is fulfilled through the "Core Program." A high degree of versatility exists within the "Core Program" making it relatively simple to adapt programs to meet individual differences. The fulfillment of these individualized programs should satisfy the hopes, aspirations, and physical needs of each participant.

As stated previously, our intent is to assist in producing "high levels of conditioning" through the use of the "Core Programs." Stop! Do not be frightened off by the phrase, "high levels of conditioning." If this phrase brings forth visions of pain, torture, and periods of extreme boredom, understand that we recognize and abide by the principle that each of us has our own "starting point."

Therefore, we recommend initial activity levels based upon the physical capabilities and readiness of the individual. Let us begin our adventure into the "Core Program," the *Golden Triangle of Activities*.

Program Experience I—Flexibility through static stretching

Program Experience II—Cardio-respiratory efficiency through aerobic activity

Program Experience III—Muscular strength and endurance through progressive resistance activity

Make these program experiences your friends. Friends you can rely on—completely. Use them to assist you in making the following adjustments:

1. As you achieve a better understanding of "self," strive for a lifetime balance of "flexibility," "Cardio-respiratory Efficiency," and "Muscular Strength and Endurance."

    For example, if you lack flexibility in certain parts of the body, put emphasis on those articulations or if you have a high degree of overall flexibility but lack muscular strength, emphasize the development of strength in your activity program. Develop a balance in these critical areas of fitness. Once this is achieved, strive throughout life to maintain a balance in the "Golden Triangle."

2. Establish regularity by including physical activity as a "way of life" but if you should regress, use these programs to renew your interest.

3. If you should experience illness, use these programs during the convalescent period.

4. If an incapacitating injury should occur, use these programs during the post-therapeutic period.
5. If a particular sport should become your activity outlet, use these programs to develop and reinforce the qualities so necessary to become more highly-skilled. These activities are the foundation for entering into the exciting world of sport and competition.
6. An emphasis on the virtues of any one particular sport or activity would be counter-productive. There exists a broad spectrum of sports activities available to all. The sport one pursues is both relevant and worthwhile so long as the individual remains active.

The activities within the "Golden Triangle" are exceptions to the above. They are basic physical activities that become ends in themselves. Each will lead to manifold benefits, both physical and psychological.

Injury Prevention Through Preventive Maintenance

The development of an optimal level of flexibility—cardio-respiratory capacity and muscular strength/endurance tends to provide the potential for more efficient and meaningful movement when an injury situation is imminent.

Increased flexibility plays a part in the prevention of injury by allowing a greater range of motion before stretching or tearing of muscle and connective tissue.

Improved cardio-respiratory capacity will reduce the number of instances in which individuals must participate while in an overly fatigued state. In a fatigued state we are more susceptible to injury because we are apt to react more slowly and be less alert.

In sports participation ankle, knee and shoulder joints are the most frequent sites for injuries which cause disability and loss of playing time. Strengthening the muscles that support these joints is one way to increase the stability of these joints. Recent scientific studies also indicate that habitual conditioning programs lead to a significant increase of strength of ligaments and tendons surrounding and protecting the joints in the body. This additional strength in ligaments and tendons will also add to joint stability. In addition optimal levels of muscular endurance provides the ability to sustain activity for longer periods, helping to delay the onset of fatigue.

Selected References

Rarick, G. L. Competitive sports for young boys: Controversial issues. *Medicine and Science in Sports,* 1969, 1, 1981–184.

Bandura, A. Social learning theory. Englewood Cliffs, N.J.: Prentice Hall, 1977.

Coopersmith, S. The antecedents of self-esteem. San Francisco: Freeman, 1967.

Scanlan, T. K. The effects of success—Failure on the perceptions of threat in a competitive situations. *Research Quarterly,* 1977, 48, 144–153.

Michenen, J. A. Sports in America. New York: Random House, 1976.

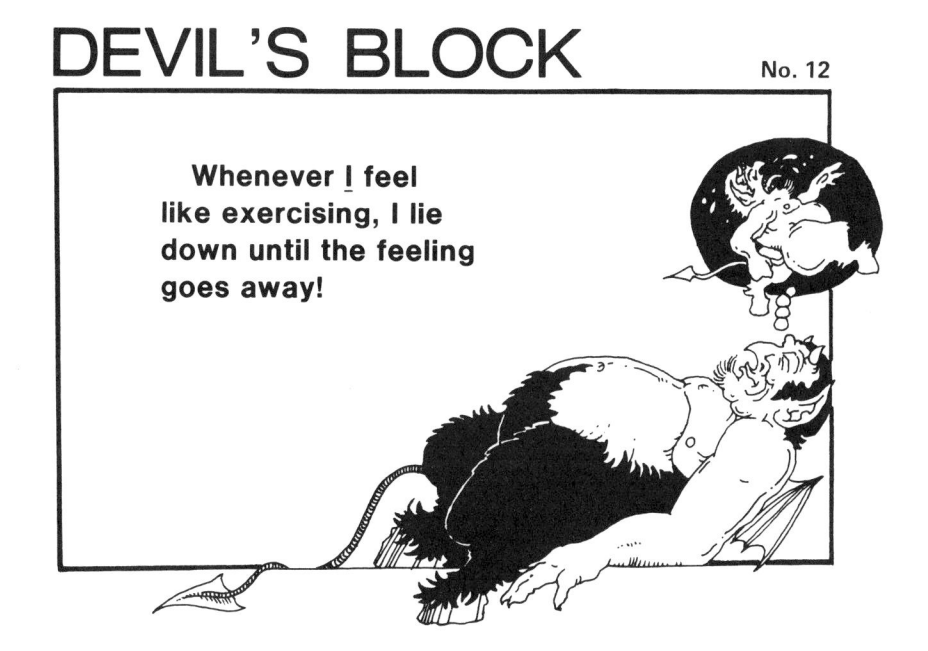

DEVIL'S BLOCK No. 12

Whenever I feel like exercising, I lie down until the feeling goes away!

13
FLEXIBILITY METHOD OF CONDITIONING

Plato once remarked, "The most beautiful motion is that which accomplishes the greatest result with the least amount of effort." The development of flexibility will bring forth this type of motion in which energy will be preserved, the onset of fatigue will be impeded, and movement will become graceful.

The development and maintenance of flexibility, regardless of age, is a simple process that may require only a few minutes of stretching each week. The price of ignoring this essential component of conditioning can be high. The resultant loss of range of motion, due to shortened muscles and tendons, could over a period of time accompany bursitis and calcium deposits restricting movement.

The onset of arthritic and rheumatic pain, with the possibility of permanent injury, may result when there is a lack of effort to maintain flexibility. Most people remain unimpressed until they become afflicted with these medical abnormalities. When this occurs, stretching and various movement forms often are recommended as therapy. Stretching to increase and maintain suppleness of muscle and joints can be a significant force in the prevention of abnormalities.

The individual whose muscles and joints are flexible can anticipate the following:

1. An intensity of performance with less chance of injury.
2. The application of full range of motion in performance of motor tasks.
3. Improved athletic potential by providing a greater range of motion in the application of muscular strength.
4. Economy of effort in the performance of skill.

Flexibility is a relative measure. It is specific to each joint; the right shoulder articulation may have limited flexibility, while the left shoulder may allow a high degree of motion. This implies that we should develop a working knowledge of stretching movements which affect all of the major articulations. The exercise program should then be geared to provide a balance of flexibility throughout the body.

The program should consist of a concentrated effort to increase the length of stretch each day. The stretching of a muscle must be accomplished slowly and the lengthening process should stop when pain is first perceived. The total stretching time should last a minimum of ten to thirty seconds.

An interesting mental exercise can add a new dimension to the flexibility program. Try this! During the exercise, conclude the lengthening process when pain is first perceived. At this precise point, concentrate on the area stretched. Sustain the stretch for twenty or thirty seconds and you will soon observe the easing of pain and its eventual disappearance which enables you to stretch further. The key is intensity of concentration. Daily stretching programs may last as little as three to five minutes and should reach each of the major joints.

Program Experience I, as depicted in the following pages, offers everyone the opportunity to perfect a well-balanced flexibility program.

PROGRAM EXPERIENCE I

These movements are designed to promote and maintain flexibility of body articulations and to stretch all muscle groups without undue strain.

All physical activities should be preceded by flexibility movements.

Become familiar with them because they are the stepping stone to all other activity. These movements can be of benefit in any of the following situations:

1. The eye-opener early in the morning.
2. The concluding activity of the day.
3. As a means of relieving tension accumulated during the day.
4. As a warm-up before entering participation in other sport activities.
5. As a warm-down at the conclusion of a progressive-resistance workout.
6. As a method of therapy during convalescence.

The following ten stretching movements (Torsion Ten) constitutes your *"Program Experience I."* Develop proficiency in their execution as they are the stepping stone to all activity.

General Directions for the "Torsion Ten"

Stretching exercises should emphasize *plastic* deformation, which is a permanent increase in the length of muscle. This goal must be accomplished without physically tearing the connective tissues involved. Ballastic stretching or high-force stretching does not enhance plastic deformation, therefore, it should not be used. High-force stretching may also weaken muscle tissue resulting in possible muscle rupture.

1. Strive to retain proper position throughout the entire movement.
2. Focus concentration on the area of the body being stretched.
3. Stretch slowly and methodically—avoiding quick movement.—"Static, low-force stretching."
4. At no time should pain be experienced. Pain may indicate tissue tearing and represent regression in the program.
5. Attempt to increase stretching ability in each workout period. Learn to stretch by how you feel—not by forcing the stretch beyond your capabilities.

6. As a warmup for specific sports—after the over-all stretching routine, emphasis should then be placed on those muscles most likely to sustain stretch injuries and on those most frequently used in the particular activity.

1. **'Good Morning'** (Hamstring—Lower Back)

Standing Position

a. Stand erect, legs straight, with feet together.
b. Reach down and grasp ankles.
c. Attempt to touch your nose to the knee area.
d. The goal is to be able to place your head and face on your knee area while your knees are locked.
e. Hold the stretch for ten seconds.

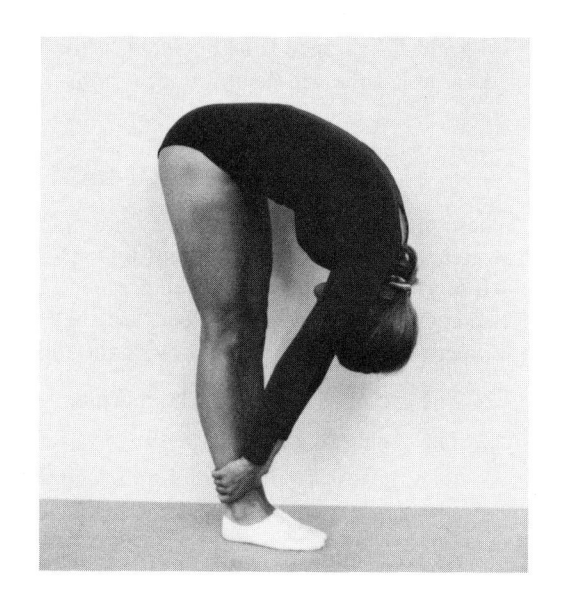

2. **'Leaning Tower'** (Achilles—Gastrocnemius)

Standing Position

a. Stand two to three feet from a wall with feet flat on floor.
b. Support upper body with hands on wall—arms extended.
c. Flex arm while leaning toward wall with pelvis—keeping feet flat on floor.
d. Hold the stretch for ten seconds.

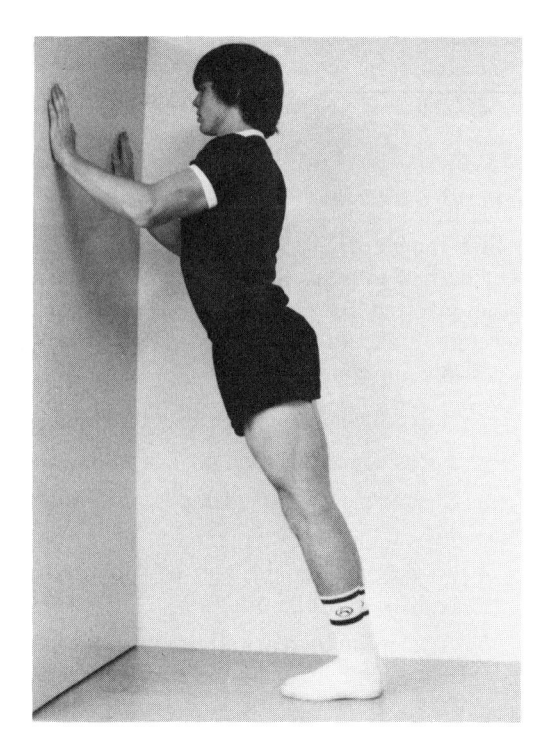

3. **'Swinger'** (Lateral Trunk—Back)

Standing Position

   a. Feet apart, lock knees and keep feet pointed straight ahead.
   b. Hold hips in a forward position. Do not rotate hips as the upper body rotates.
   c. Keep arms and hands up and to the side in a lightly flexed, relaxed position.
   d. Rotate body to the left by turning head, shoulders and arms with the trunk. Follow the complete turn with your eyes watching the hands.
   e. Reverse by rotating to the right.
   f. Hold the full stretch at each side for three seconds before reversing direction.
   g. Perform five repetitions to each side.

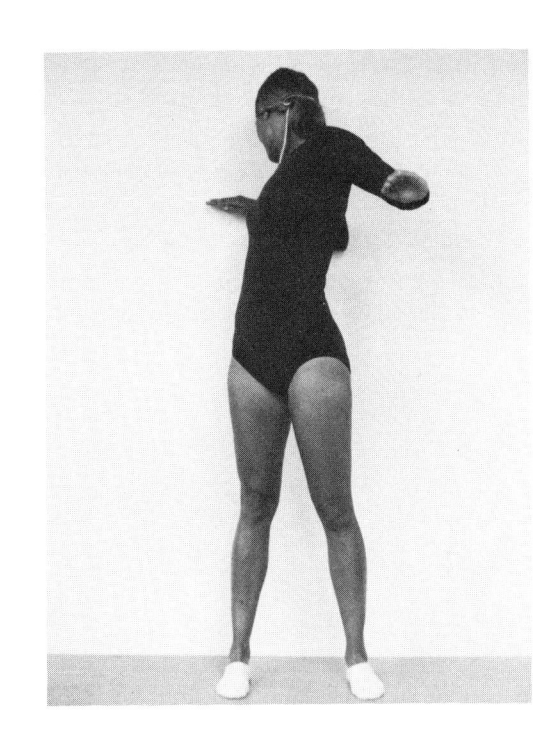

4. **'Hurdler'** (Hamstring—Calf—Trunk—Quadriceps)

Sitting Position (Hurdlers)

   a. Left leg straight—knee locked—right leg flexed with the foot drawn towards the buttock and knee.
   b. Begin by reaching for lead foot with both hands—hold for ten seconds.
   c. Lean gradually back trying to touch head to floor—hold for ten seconds.
   d. Alternate position.

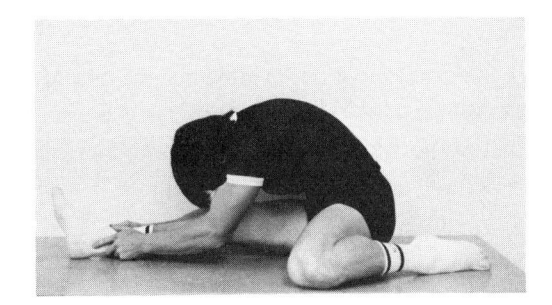

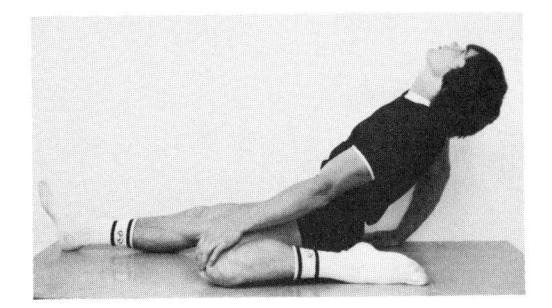

5. **'Tailor'** (Groin)

Sitting Position

   a. Sit with both knees flexed—soles of the feet together.
   b. Grasp ankles, draw heels into groin.
   c. Ease the knees downward with pressure from the elbows attempting to touch the floor.
   d. Hold for ten seconds.

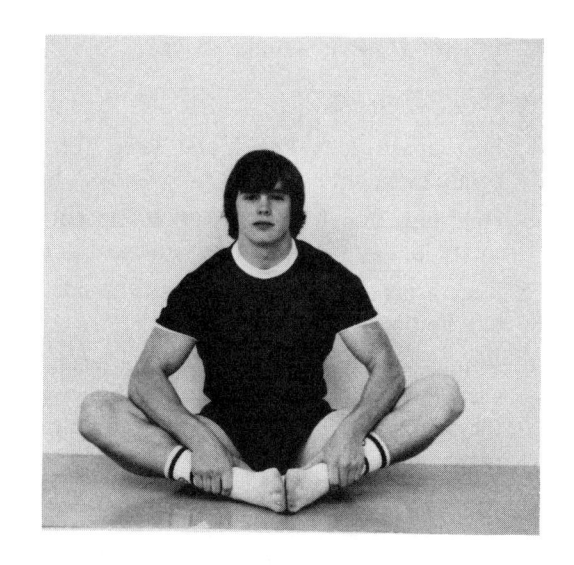

6. **'Lunger'** (Groin and Hip Flexer)

Standing Position

   a. Right foot in front pointing straight ahead while the left foot is back slanted sideways.
   b. Keep back foot flat to allow for maximum stretch.
   c. Lean forward and down with weight.
   d. Keep back straight and head up.
   e. Hold stretch for ten seconds.
   f. Alternate.

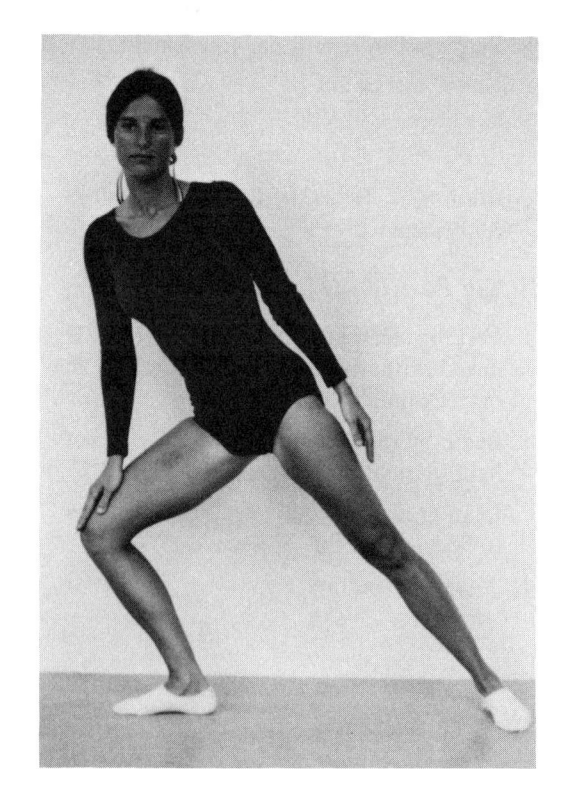

7. 'Swaying Palm' (Quadriceps)

Kneeling Position

a. Knees slightly spread—legs behind the body with toes pointed to the rear.
b. The back and neck are straight.
c. Reach back and grasp ankles for support during exercise.
d. Lean back slowly, lowering upper body toward floor.
e. The objective is to eventually touch your head to the floor while lower legs remain flat.
f. Stretch as far as you can and hold for ten seconds.

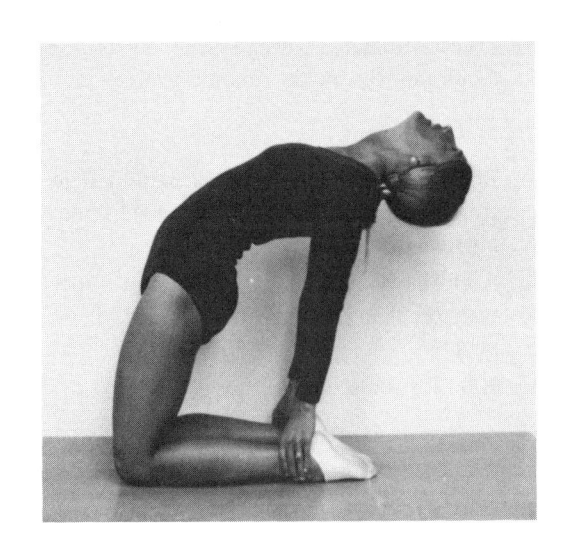

8. 'Side Winder' (Hips—Lower Back)

Supine Position

a. Keep legs straight, feet together, knees locked with toes pointed forward.
b. Arms extended to side.
c. Lift left leg up straight and hold briefly—keep knee locked—point toe upward.
d. Swing leg over and touch toes to opposite hand—hold three seconds before returning to starting position.
e. Repeat stretching to opposite side.

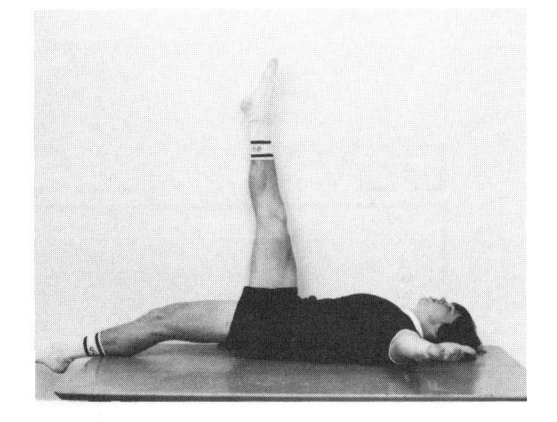

9. 'The Jackknife' (back—Hamstring)

Supine Position

a. Body fully extended—arms at the side—palms down.
b. Keep legs straight with feet together—toes pointed forward, knees locked.
c. Flex at the waist and lift legs over head.
d. Touch toes to floor.
e. Hold for ten seconds—return slowly to starting position.

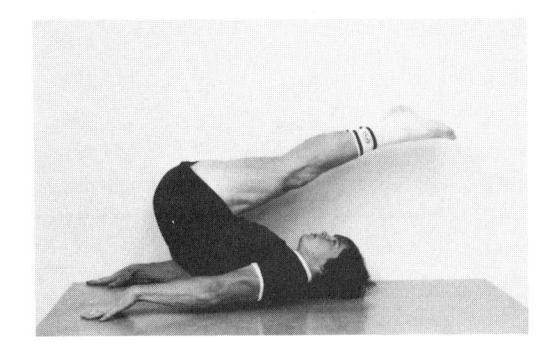

10. **'The Swimmer'** (Lower Back—Vertebrae Column—Buttocks—Shoulders)

Prone Position

a. Body fully extended—arms extended to front—legs together—knees locked—toes pointed to rear.
b. Arch the body lifting the chin and upper body off floor, along with legs as high as possible.
c. Hold for ten seconds.

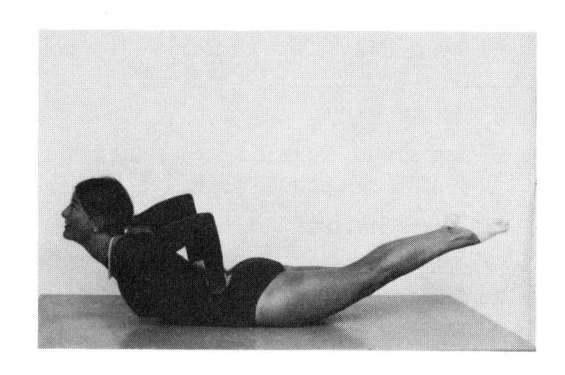

Selected References

Anderson, R.: The perfect pre-run stretching routine. *Runners World* 13 (5): 56, 1978.
DeVries, H.: Evaluation of static stretching procedures for improvement of flexibility. *Research Quarterly.*, 33:222–229, 1962.
Leighton, J.: Flexibility charcteristics of four specialized skill groups of college athletes. *Arch. Phys. Med. Rehabil.*, 38: 24–28, 1957.
Ryan, A. J.: Yoga and Fitness. *J. Health Phys. Educ. Recr.* 42(2): 26; 1971.
Wickstrom, R. L.: Weight training and flexibility. *J. Health, Phys. Educ. Recr.* 34 (2): 61, 1963.

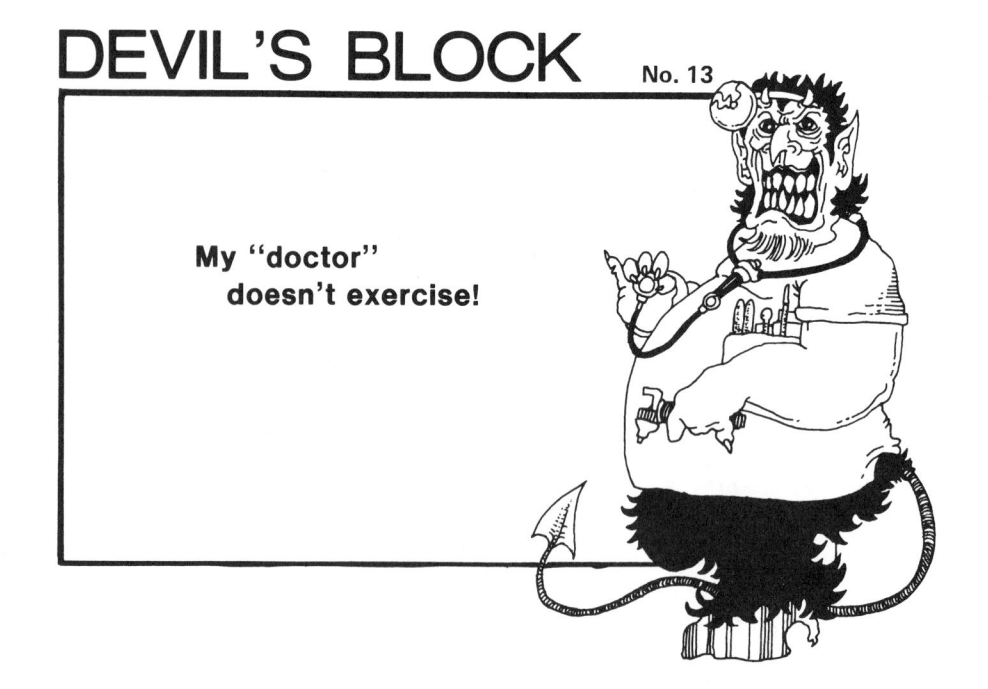

DEVIL'S BLOCK No. 13

My "doctor" doesn't exercise!

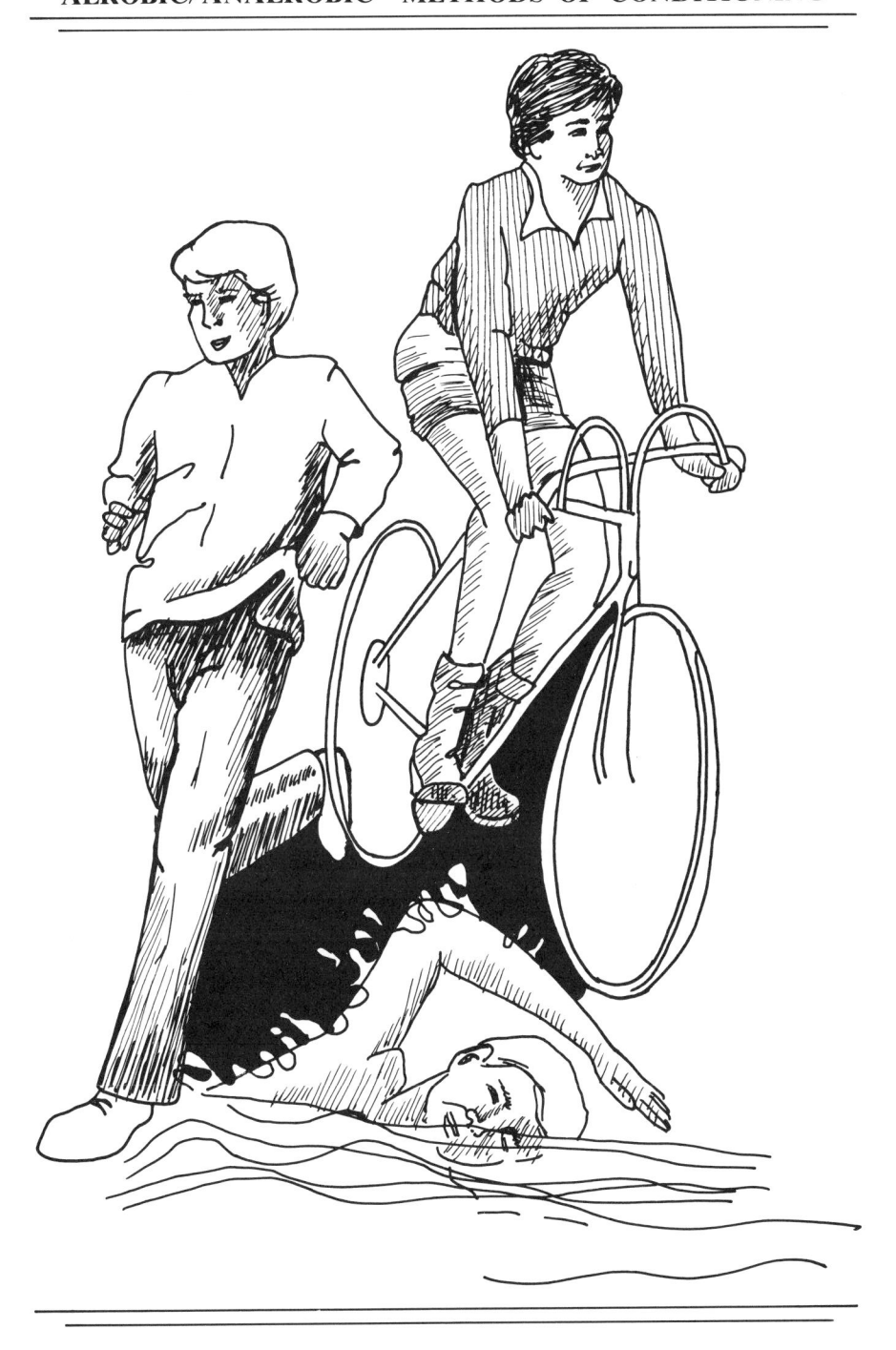

AEROBIC/ANAEROBIC—METHODS OF CONDITIONING

14
AEROBIC/ANAEROBIC METHOD OF CONDITIONING

The foundation of virtually all conditioning programs is the capacity of the cardio-respiratory system to endure. This is basic to all activities in which stamina is a critical factor. Aerobic (with air) exercise is the most efficient means of improving the capacity and functioning of the heart, lungs and circulatory system. Aerobic training forces the heart rate to increase and maintain levels in which training effects result.

Anaerobic (without air) exercise stimulates a quick increase in the heart rate, which unfortunately produces insurmountable oxygen deficit resulting in a cessation or reduction in activity. This form of training exerts its greatest influence on the cardio-respiratory system after the individual has reached adequate conditioning levels. For this reason we recommend aerobic training for those who are about to begin a personal fitness program.

Aerobic training is continuous and can be maintained for long periods of time without producing an intolerable oxygen deficit. Long-distance runners often run continuously for six hours and more. This system of continuous cardio-respiratory stimulation unleashes the "training effect" in which wondrous physiological changes occur. The lungs begin processing more oxygen with less effort, the heart grows stronger, pumping an increased blood volume with fewer strokes, and the capillary bed expands supplying more blood to muscle tissue. In short, you are improving your body's capacity to gather and deliver oxygen to the tissue cells where it combines with foodstuffs in producing energy. Consequently, your endurance capacity is enhanced.

We recommend jogging, swimming and cycling as the exercise mediums. These three forms of exercise are practical, relatively inexpensive, and lead to a quick elicitation of a multitude of training effects.

A wise man once said, "I have two doctors; my left leg and my right." This may be an overgeneralization, but true nonetheless.

If you lack the ability to jog make walking your workout. As the legs gain strength and breathing becomes easier the pace should increase. Flat terrain is advised until fitness levels are reached. Walking can then be interspersed with light jogging. Eventually, you will be able to discontinue walking and jog for extended periods. If weather restricts you from going out-of-doors, running in place serves a similar purpose. To bring forth the training effects, persist in running each day. Little time is required, as the minimal duration of each workout may be twelve minutes. Once you break through the training barrier of mental and physical discomforts, you will look forward to exercise as an elixir and running will become pleasurable.

JOGGING FOR THE BEGINNER

At the onset of jogging, it is best to jog every other day. If the beginner jogs every day, the chances of developing foot or leg problems increase. After a period of time, the body develops an acceptable level of condition and the number of days in which one jogs may be increased. Other aspects of the "Golden Triangle," including flexibility and resistive exercises may be performed on off days. If this initial program is too difficult, replace some of the jogging with walking or reduce the total distance covered each day. Be sure to always start each workout with flexibility exercises and end it by tapering off with a walk for at least several minutes. These procedures will help reduce any muscle soreness that might occur. Once this introductory period of jogging is completed, a person should be experienced enough to design a regular exercise program to fit their own needs, schedule, facilities and interests.

What is jogging? Jogging is a form of exercise that consists either of alternate walking and running (interval training) at a slow-to-moderate pace or running at a slow steady pace. The amount and intensity of exercise performed while jogging may be varied by regulating the total distance covered, the ratio of walking to running and the pace of running.

Why jogging? Jogging is of particular value since it provides the opportunity for a graduated program of physical activity that can be performed by most people regardless of age, sex, or level of physical fitness. It does not require much in the way of special skills, equipment, facilities or supervision nor does it require locating teammates or opponents as do many sports or games. Jogging is extremely valuable for many inactive adults since it permits gradual conditioning without the risk of traumatic injuries.

How to jog? There is no one correct way to jog. Just as everyone walks in a slightly different way, their manner of jogging will also vary. Here are some general suggestions to follow which will make jogging more enjoyable and will help reduce any muscular or joint soreness that might occur.

1. Keep the back straight while maintaining a natural and comfortable posture. Hold the head up and focus the eyes about 5 yards in front.

2. The arms should be held slightly away from the body and bent at the elbows so that the elbow and hand are approximately the same distance from the ground. The arms should be moved in a rhythmical forward and backward pattern with little or no sideward movement. Occasional shaking and relaxing the arms and shoulders while running will help reduce the tightness that sometimes develop. Periodically taking several deep breaths helps to foster relaxation.

3. Foot position and plant is an important part of a successful jogging technique. There are several acceptable techniques. One is to land first on the heel of the foot slightly before the bottom of the foot touches, then rock forward and take off from the ball of the foot on the next step . If this procedure is found to be uncomfortable or unnatural, try landing on the entire bottom of the foot all at once with most of the weight on the ball of the foot. An attempt should be made to avoid landing on the ball of the foot because this will create unnecessary foot and leg soreness.

4. Regardless of what method is used, keep each step short by letting the foot strike the ground beneath the knee instead of projecting it out in front. The stride will shorten as the pace or rate of running decreases.

5. Remember to exhale forcefully and let the air come in naturally. Some people like to develop a rhythm in breathing by alternating exhalation and inhalation every two or three steps.
6. Any individual who becomes unusually tired or uncomfortable while jogging should take it easy, slow down, walk or stop.

Jogging is only one of several activities that may be effectively employed in the improvement and maintenance of cardio-respiratory capacity.

BICYCLING

Cycling is similar to jogging in that the legs are utilized in a pumping motion. Because of this fact, bicycling can be approached in much the same manner as jogging. Training effects including increased cardio-respiratory endurance quickly appear when the training program reaches appropriate levels of intensity, duration and frequency. Replacing the car with a bicycle whenever possible can make a contribution toward energy conservation as well as promote high levels of fitness and positive health.

How to bicycle? Basic guidelines for success and enjoyment in the sport of bicycling.

1. Exercise descrimination in bicycle selection. Select a bike that fits you and your needs. Consider the type and height of seat, style of bike (racer or recreation), weight of frame and gear potential.
2. Pedal exclusively with the ball of the foot.
3. Ideally, the seat should be adjusted so when a leg is fully extended, the heel rests on the bottom pedal. This creates a slight flexing of the knee when the ball of the foot is placed properly on the pedal, ready to initiate the pumping action.

Why cycling? Cycling can make a significant contribution toward physical fitness. Riding a minimum of 12 miles per hour on a level course, for at least 30 minutes, three times a week will result in the development of excellent muscular strength and endurance of the lower extremities. Vigorous competitive cycling will promote increases in strength and endurance in the arms, abdomen, chest, shoulders, back and neck muscles.

The most important contribution of cycling lies in its potential to produce cardio respiratory training effects. The key to insure the production of cardio respiratory fitness is to constantly monitor the heart rate. The heart rate should always equal the threshold of training (target rate). Simply stop the bike, look at your watch and measure your heart rate for 10 seconds. Multiply your heart rate by six. If the product is under your target, increase the intensity by peddling harder. As was stated earlier continuous aerobic activity can be extremely effective in reducing the incidence of degenerative cardio-vascular disease. Bicycling can play an important role in the achievement of this goal.

SWIMMING

Swimming is an activity universally endorsed by the medical profession, since virtually every mucle is utilized as we push and pull ourselves through liquid resistance.

A fitness through swimming program can help regain some of the vitality lost by living a sedentary life. Along with the enhancement of fitness there is a great deal of fun which may be derived from swimming. For those who have never learned the art of swimming, it is never too late to acquire a degree of proficiency in the skills necessary to enjoy swimming. In terms of water safety and fulfillment of fitness, participation in swimming is invaluable. Time and effort put forth to achieve a higher level of proficiency will reap many rewards.

How to begin swimming? A fitness through swimming program based on three principles:

Principle #1—Swimming is not a high injury activity. However pulled muscles and undue strain can result from unaccustomed exercise. A routine of flexibility exercises in which the body temperature is elevated and muscles are stretched should be completed before entering the water.

Principle #2—A progressive program of swimming eventually leading to vigorous swimming can help to lower the pulse-rate, improve breath-holding ability, improve strength and endurance of the arms and legs, and reduce body fat. A program of swimming should be initiated gradually. Progressively build up the tolerance to swim. The frequency and duration in which you swim will influence how rapid the advancement will be. Daily activity is best but significant gain can be attained by swimming two or three times a week.

Principle #3—The muscular and cardio-respiratory systems respond when they are taxed beyond the load they are accustomed to. Add intensity, placing additional demands upon the body by attempting to swim the same distance in less time.

Why swimming? To be successful, swimming like any other form of activity should be pleasurable with the fitness benefits as the by-product. It is important to remember that we must give ourselves a chance to develop skill (serve the apprentice period), and to break through the exercise barrier. Activities which at first appear to be distasteful may then become highly pleasurable experiences. Give yourself a chance!

Establish realistic goals. An eventual goal to strive for would be to swim 500 yards (20 lengths of a 25-yard pool equals 500 yards). If certain muscles become tired as you increase your distance, try changing the swimming stroke. This will bring different muscles into use and give some relief to the muscles which were under stress.

A second objective should be to swim the same distance using just one stroke. The switch to the use of one stroke should be as gradual as the original buildup to added distance. The stroke used should be either the breast stroke or the crawl stroke, which require rhythmical breathing between each stroke. The added stress imposed by breathing between strokes will help to improve respiratory efficiency. Eventually a level of skill and fitness will be reached and one should be able to swim five hundred yards with little difficulty.

SUMMARY

Jogging, cycling and swimming should be altered in duration, frequency and intensity in response to any unpleasant sensations, both physiological and psychological. An individual should not be exposed to a great deal of discomfort until ability to tolerate stress has been heightened. We should prevent overdoing any form of activity to a point where it may become so distasteful that it is dreaded or eventually eliminated from our daily life.

You may select one of these training activities exclusively, or you may alternate them to provide a change of pace. For example, jog one day and cycle the next. We are limiting the activity in this area to jogging, cycling and swimming since they are convenient and effective activities for the purpose of developing and maintaining cardio-respiratory capacity. The principles of exercise related to increasing tolerance, overload and progression can be reasonably well applied and controlled.

Techniques of Training

There are a number of techniques of organizing training programs. The selection of a specific type of training depends, in large measure, upon the goals one desires to accomplish. For the sake of simplification, we can view these goals in the following categories:

1. Maximal speed.
2. Movement efficiency.
3. Stress tolerance.
4. Recovery time.
5. Cardio-respiratory endurance.

These areas can be influenced by applying the following training methods to the aerobic/anaerobic activities of jogging, swimming and cycling.

(A) *Distance Training*—"Putting in the Miles"—In this form of conditioning, the individual trains by logging great distances each day at considerably less than maximal speed. The major benefits of distance training fall into the areas of cardio-respiratory conditioning and movement efficiency. This training regimen seems to be the cornerstone of most athletic programs, for those who compete in distance events and those involved in personal fitness programs.

(B) *Interval Training*—Most sprint and middle-distance athletes use this method of structuring their training programs. A distance is selected for which a maximum or near-maximum effort is put forth. After finishing the exercise in an anaerobic state, the individual takes a brief rest and repeats the initial effort. These intervals of anaerobic activity followed by rest are repeated a number of times during the exercise period. Interval training can take a variety of forms. The following forms of interval training have been found to be of great value in the development of speed and stress tolerance.

1. *Repetition Training*—The exercise bouts are of specified distances—each interspersed with a recovery period.
2. *Fartlek*—Long periods of cruising are interspersed with bursts of maximum or near-maximum efforts. Emphasis is on changing tempos of speed. Distances traveled at these varying speeds are irregular.
3. *Relay Training*—A team of two to four individuals perform a continuous relay in which one person is active while the others are resting.
4. *Resistance Training*—The exercises are performed with additional resistance. A few examples are: riding a bike with a passenger, running up hill, running in sand, and swimming while holding or pulling additional resistance.

5. *Pyramid Training*—The distance logged in any one training session is arranged in ascending or descending lengths.
6. *Forced Intensity*—The individual expends maximum effort for a short period of time (twenty seconds) and takes an extremely brief recovery period of approximately five seconds. These intervals are repeated, but because of the extreme intensity of exercise, this type of training can only last from three to five minutes.

(C) *Circuit Training*—This system is based upon organizing a series of exercise stations in a manner allowing the individual to pass from one station to the next. The circuit may be completed with fixed recovery periods or with no rest between each station. The versatility of the circuit is unlimited depending upon one's imagination in setting it up. This technique of training forces the heart rate up and allows it to maintain a high mean rate throughout the circuit. Circuit training is excellent in promoting motor efficiency, aerobic benefits and muscular endurance.

PROGRAM EXPERIENCE II

The following programs are examples of the many possibilities of organizing aerobic/anaerobic systems of training (jogging, cycling, and swimming).

A. *Distance Training*

1. Swimming—long distance at aerobic speeds
2. Jogging—long distance at aerobic speeds
3. Cycling—long distance at aerobic speeds

B. *Forms of Interval Training*

1. Repetition Training

    100-yard dash—maximum speed
    30 second rest

    100-yard dash—maximum speed
    30 second rest

    100-yard dash—maximum speed
    30 second rest

    100-yard dash—maximum speed
    30 second rest

2. *Fartlek Training*—The emphasis in Fartlek Training is on changing the tempo of speed. This example should not imply fixed distances. The distances and tempo are constantly changing.

Jog—440 yards
Sprint—100 yards
Jog—880 yards
Sprint—220 yards
Jog—1 mile
Sprint—40 yards
Jog—880 yards
Sprint—50 yards
Jog—1 mile.

3. *Pyramid Training*

25-yard freestyle—1 minute rest
50-yard freestyle—1 minute rest
75-yard freestyle—1 minute rest
100-yard freestyle—1 minute rest
125-yard freestyle—1 minute rest
100-yard freestyle—1 minute rest
75-yard freestyle—1 minute rest
50-yard freestyle—1 minute rest
25-yard freestyle—1 minute rest

C. *Circuit Training*

Example 1—track

Station

1. Good Morning Stretch
2. Twenty Push-ups
3. Ten Squat Jumps
4. 440-Yard Jog
5. Thirty Sit-ups
6. 100-Yard Dash
7. Tailor Stretch
8. Fifteen Squat Thrusts
9. Hurdler Stretch
10. 880-Yard Jog

Example 2—swimming

Station

1. Freestyle 25 Yards
2. Seven Push-ups
3. Tread Water 30 Second
4. Fifteen Sit-ups
5. Two Lengths Freestyle
6. Ten Squat Thrusts
7. Two Lengths Backstroke
8. Five Pull-ups
9. Jackknife Stretch
10. Freestyle 25 Yards

C. *Circuit Training*

Example 3

DIAGRAM OF A CIRCUIT-INTERVAL COURSE

Circuit training is a program of timed exercises on an organized obstacle course. The object is to complete the course as quickly as possible while still doing the individual exercises correctly.

Versatility is the beauty of circuit training for any aspect of total fitness can be stressed.

Circuit training can demand a short, concentrated effort and the conditioned person will receive maximum benefit from the program in a minimum amount of time. However, if run improperly, circuit training may place a great strain on the deconditioned person. Initiating a strenuous program without being sufficiently prepared and accustomed to moderate amounts of stress could be extremely undesirable. Remember, any program of activity must be approached gradually and tolerance should be built up progressively. This is especially important in circuit training.

Used correctly, the circuit can be adjusted to meet the needs of the deconditioned individual as well as the individual who is an outstanding example of physical perfection. The following chart is flexible in that; the time interval between each station; the repetitions or duration at each station; the intensity of each exercise; can all be adjusted. The adaptations are dependent upon the individuals goals and level of condition.

Summary

Program Experience II triggers aerobic and anaerobic benefits in the cardio-respiratory system and endurance increases in the muscular system. Relaxation and movement efficiency also result from this type of training. For the super-sapien this fashion of conditioning offers the greatest advantages for more healthful daily living.

CIRCUIT TRAINING—EXAMPLE #3
DIAGRAM FOR CIRCUIT-INTERVAL COURSE

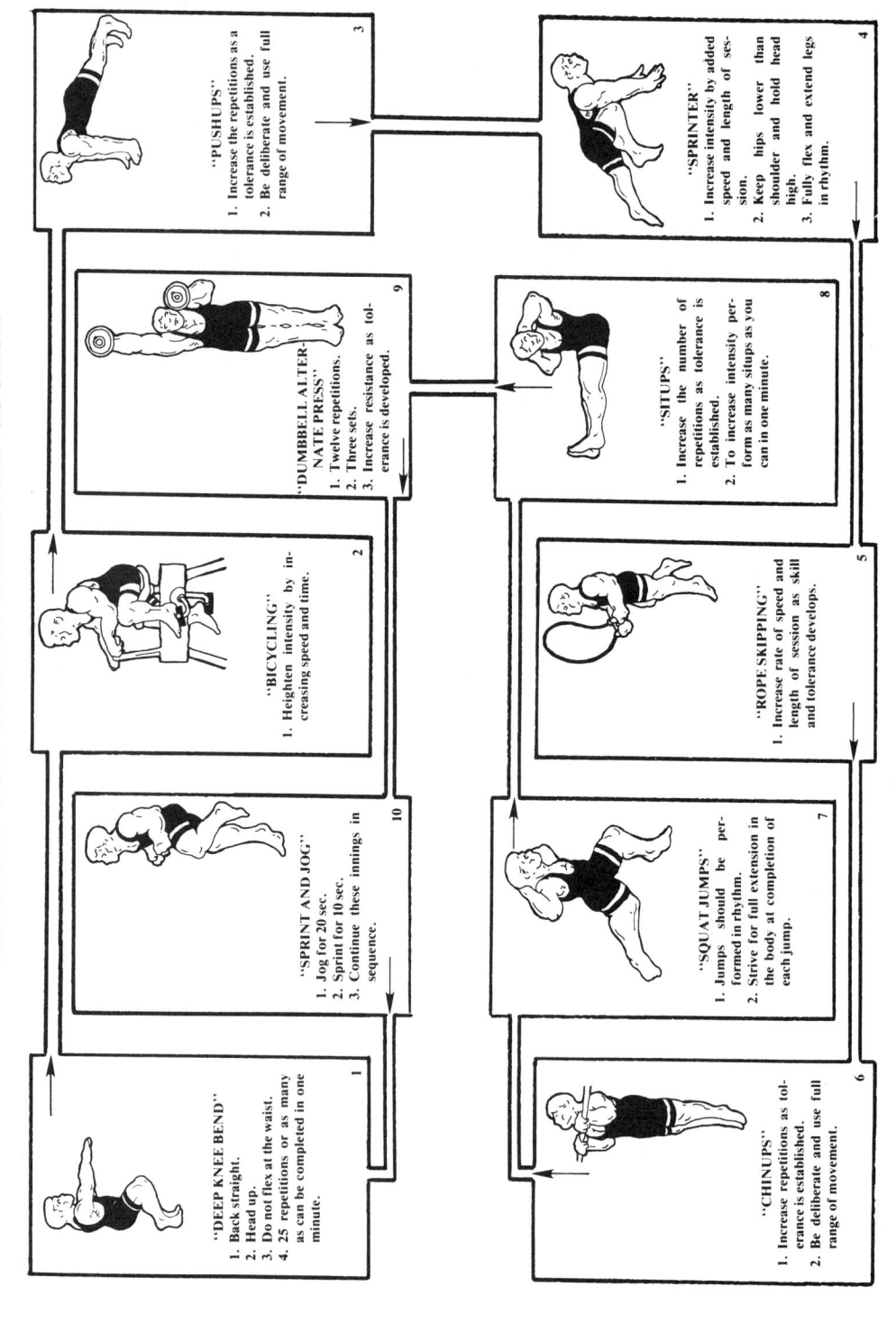

"DEEP KNEE BEND"
1. Back straight.
2. Head up.
3. Do not flex at the waist.
4. 25 repetitions or as many as can be completed in one minute.

"BICYCLING"
1. Heighten intensity by increasing speed and time.

"PUSHUPS"
1. Increase the repetitions as a tolerance is established.
2. Be deliberate and use full range of movement.

"SPRINTER"
1. Increase intensity by added speed and length of session.
2. Keep hips lower than shoulder and hold head high.
3. Fully flex and extend legs in rhythm.

"ROPE SKIPPING"
1. Increase rate of speed and length of session as skill and tolerance develops.

"CHINUPS"
1. Increase repetitions as tolerance is established.
2. Be deliberate and use full range of movement.

"SQUAT JUMPS"
1. Jumps should be performed in rhythm.
2. Strive for full extension in the body at completion of each jump.

"SITUPS"
1. Increase the number of repetitions as tolerance is established.
2. To increase intensity perform as many situps as you can in one minute.

"DUMBBELL ALTERNATE PRESS"
1. Twelve repetitions.
2. Three sets.
3. Increase resistance as tolerance is developed.

"SPRINT AND JOG"
1. Jog for 20 sec.
2. Sprint for 10 sec.
3. Continue these innings in sequence.

Selected References

Bransford, P. R., and Howley, E. T. Oxygen cost of running in trained and untrained men and women. *Medicine and Science in Sports,* 1977, 9, 41–44.

Costill, D. L. Physiology of marathon running. *Journal of the American Medical Association,* 1972; 221, 1024–1029.

Dolgener, F. A. Prediction of maximum aerobic power in untrained females. *Research Quarterly,* 1978, 49, 20–27.

Faulker, J. A. Physiology of swimming. *Research Quarterly,* 1966, 37, 41–54.

Henry, F., DeMoor, J. Metabolic efficiency of exercise in relation to work load at constant speed. *Journal of Applied Physiology.* 1950, 2, 481–287.

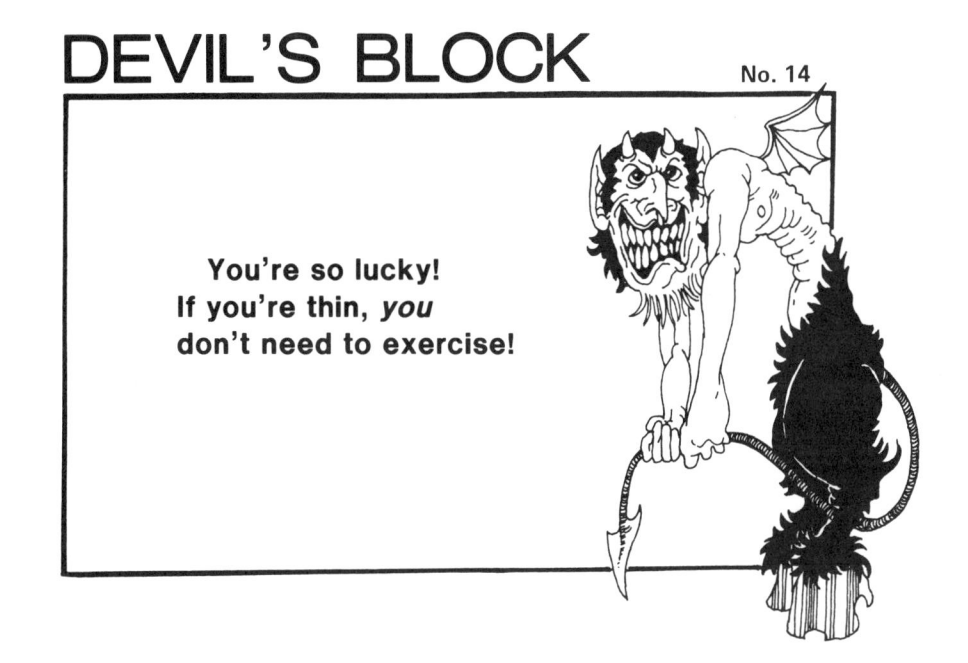

DEVIL'S BLOCK No. 14

You're so lucky! If you're thin, *you* don't need to exercise!

15
PROGRESSIVE RESISTANCE METHOD OF CONDITIONING

For centuries, forms of moving resistance have resulted in the development of muscular mass and strength. The fact that our body grows larger and heavier as we mature forces us to move a greater resistance and thus, we gain strength naturally. This is nature's example of progressive resistance. Progressive resistance exercise is the most expedient method for the improvement of muscular strength, endurance and tonus.

Until recently, most people believed the only value of progressive resistance exercise was in the development of the "professional strongman." They held contempt for weight training, citing "muscle boundness" as an adverse effect of increased muscle mass. As professionals began to study this area, they discovered the amazing potential for strength and muscle mass development, and ironically found that progressive resistance workouts had a positive effect on agility. Today, coaches have included some variety of resistance exercise into virtually all sport activities.

Improving muscular tonus and strength has an effect upon the size and shape of the muscle. This improves appearance and alters body shape, resulting in a more pleasing body symmetry.

The term, "Progressive Resistance Exercise" implies a logical sequence in the amount of resistance encountered by a muscle or muscle group throughout a range of motion. The underlying principle of progressive resistance training is to overload the muscle, exposing it to increased work loads. As muscle strength and endurance are promoted, the resistance must also increase if the "overload" principle is to remain in effect.

There are many techniques, innovations and forms of equipment available for the conduction of progressive resistive programs. Traditionally, the barbell and dumbbell have been the mainstays of these systems. We have listed below some of the equipment and devices that are capable of eliciting training effects:

1. Barbell and Dumbbell—usually cast iron, steel, or plastic filled with water or sand.
2. Multistationed machines—in some of these devices up to eighteen people can be working at the same time. A number of these machines utilize isokenetic principles.
3. Expanders—based on springs or bands of rubber that are stretched.
4. Devices utilizing cams and gears.

Each of us will realize individual gains at different rates and stages. Such factors as individual potential, effort expended, time devoted, personal limitations and attitudes are all factors influencing progress. Successful muscular development occurs only as a result of use, for disuse means muscle atrophy.

WEIGHT TRAINING FOR MUSCULAR STRENGTH, ENDURANCE AND POWER

Definition

Weight training is a systematic series of resistance exercises designed to promote physical development and conditioning or to rehabilitate persons who have suffered injury or illness. The term weight training is differentiated from *weight lifting* which is the practice and participation of lifting weights in competition.

Weight training is now almost universally accepted as an effective and efficient means of developing muscular strength, endurance and power. Strength is the ability to exert force in overcoming resistance and is an important component in sports performance. Muscular endurance can be thought of as the ability of the muscles to continue or persist in contraction over a period of time. Power, as used here, refers to a combination of strength and speed. It is the ability to apply strength in an "explosive" movement.

Additional Values

1. Weight training, *when performed properly,* may contribute to flexibility, the ability of the joints to move through a full range of motion. Flexibility is enhanced when opposing muscle groups are in balance and the muscles and connective tissue are of proper length and elasticity.

2. Training with weights, under certain conditions, may also contribute to another primary component of physical fitness—cardio-respiratory capacity. Such conditions require that the exercises be done rhythmically and consecutively with little or no rest in between exercise bouts.

3. A well-chosen sequence of weight training exercises, pursued regularly over a period of time can also bring about significant improvement in posture and appearance as body measurements are reapportioned and sagging body contours firmed up.

4. Weight training is particularly worthwhile in helping the physically underdeveloped person since the regimen and goals can be easily adapted to individual needs and capacities. Even the weakest and smallest student can be challenged to improve since progress can be noted in a relatively short period of time.

5. Important psychological benefits in poise, self-discipline, self-direction, and self-realization are often derived.

6. Weight training can result in a significant improvement in sports performance through increased strength, endurance and power.

7. Women have much to gain from weight training which was once looked upon as an exclusive activity for men. Progressive resistance exercises can be easily adapted to each woman's capacity, ability and needs. Most American women lack adequate strength in arms, shoulders and trunk, and could profit from a developmental routine. The fear that lifting weights will develop bulky, over-defined and heavily-muscled women has been

soundly disproved. In fact, quite the opposite occurs. A trim, firm, well-contoured figure is usually found among women who undertake regular exercise of this kind. Remember! *"Behind Every Curve is a Muscle."*

Safety Considerations

The danger of injury and accidents can be minimized if the following precautions are adopted:

1. Everyone should have a medical examination—work within your limitations.
2. Train with a partner and utilize spotters in the following movements:
    a. Bench Press
    b. Press Behind Neck
    c. Squat
    d. Pullovers
3. Warm up with the "Tortion Ten" and various body resistance movements.
4. Do not start exercises with maximal resistance, instead work up to heavy loads.
5. Breathing should consist of inhaling as resistance is being lowered or as you return to the starting position. Hold breath momentarily as exercise motion is initiated and then exhale.
6. During the first month of training, use less than maximal resistance while learning the movements allowing the joints and muscles to adjust.
7. Be sure each movement is smooth and utilize the entire range of motion. Jerky and violent movements, especially during the lowering of resistance, can result in joint injuries.
8. Strive for balanced development. Exercise the antagonist as well as the agonist muscle groups. If this is practiced, range of motion will increase. However, if balanced development does not occur, great losses of flexibility can result.
9. Do not perform any motion in which pain is experienced. This should be differentiated from the natural soreness of muscles during the adjustment period.

Program Development

The training program consists of several exercises (called lifts) which utilize either free weights or resistance machines.

Most weight training programs use the principle of repetitions and sets. "Repetitions" may be defined as the number of times a motion is repeated during a specific exercise. "Set" indicates the number of times an exercise is performed during the training session. For example, if an exercise is performed for 10 reps, 8 reps and 6 reps, three sets have been completed. The selection of exercise routines, the amount of weight used and the number of repetitions and sets performed are adjusted to the capacities and objectives of the individual.

The number and types of exercises included in most programs are selected to reach the major muscle groups in the body. We have included a brief description of the various systems of progressive resistance conditioning. Each system has certain advantages that may stimulate its adoption as a preferable means of reaching a similar goal. In order to overcome "the plateau tendency" when progress ceases in a program, alternate the activity. We recommend that the basic program be used by beginners and that one moves to advanced systems only after significant gains are realized.

(A) *Basic Program*—This program is the most universally utilized system of weight training. It consists of working out three alternate days per week, using from two to three sets for each exercise with from six to ten repetitions per set. Many variations of manipulating poundages and repetitions can be suggested:

1. Same resistance—three sets—as many repetitions as possible.
2. Lowered resistance—second and third sets—in order to maintain or increase repetitions.
3. Increased resistance—second and third sets—in order to perform less repetitions with muscular mass and strength as the goals.

(B) *Single Progressive System*—Keeping the same number of repetitions in each set and adding resistance wherever possible.

(C) *Double Progressive System*—Start with a resistance that can be handled for five or six repetitions. Continue with this resistance during each session, attempting additional repetitions until the goal of ten repetitions is accomplished. Add resistance and reduce repetitions to five or six. This is used quite often in the basic program.

(D) *Circuit Training Program*—Exercises are performed at stations using one set with a definite number of repetitions. The participant passes from one station to the next as rapidly as possible limiting any rest between exercise bouts. This forces the heart rate up and maintains the high pulse throughout the circuit so that aerobic benefits accompany the muscular strength and endurance increases. Methods of increasing the work load follow:

1. Decrease time of completing the circuit.
2. Increase number of circuits.
3. Increase number of stations.
4. Increase number of repetitions.

(E) *Light and Heavy System*—In this workout, resistance considerably lower than maximum is selected for each exercise, and eight repetitions are executed in the first set. Additional resistance is added in each set and the eight repetitions are performed again in each succeeding set, gradually diminishing until one repetition is performed. This system, used by many competitive lifters, has definite advantages in building muscular strength.

(F) *Heavy and Light System*—In this system the individual starts by using a maximum resistance that can be lifted a set number of repetitions (eight). This resistance is gradually reduced to enable the individual to perform the set number of repetitions. The procedure is continued for as long as possible. Research has shown that as the muscle is exposed to near maximal resistance in this manner for extended periods of time, strength and endurance ensues.

(G) *Supersetting*—Exercises are selected which offer resistance to the agonist and antagonist muscle groups. These are alternated for a predetermined number of sets. For example, the "curl" and "french curl" alternately stimulate the biceps and the triceps. This is extremely fatiguing and is especially useful for those interested in perfecting body symmetry.

(H) *Flushing Principle*—This system is designed so that the participant begins by exercising one end of the body such as the neck and shoulders, and progressively shifts exercise areas toward the ankles and feet. The principle of flushing has muscular endurance value since similar and assisting muscle groups remain working until the exercise pattern has progressed to a new muscle group.

(I) *Cheating Exercises*—This principle consists of lifting more resistance than the body can handle in strict form. This is accomplished by bringing into action supporting muscle groups to help move the resistance past the "sticking point." This system, when properly utilized, is excellent for building strength since the individual is exposed to maximal resistances.

(J) *Compound Exercises*—As a timesaving device, we may combine two exercises such as the reverse curl-press and the dead lift—shoulder shrug. The disadvantage here lies in the fact that the resistance is determined by the weight that can be handled in the movement in which there is less strength potential.

(K) *Peripheral Heart System*—The objective of utilizing this system is to elevate the heart rate, producing aerobic and muscular training effects. A series of from five to six exercises are selected and arranged in sequence so that a different body part is worked during each exercise. An example of a sequence might be the military press, toe raise, bent rowing, deep knee bend and curl. Each exercise is performed for six to ten repetitions and each sequence is repeated from two to five times. The intent is to limit the rest period between each exercise and sequence. This system has great aerobic potential and contributes to strength, muscular endurance and definition.

(L) *Rest Pause System*—Developing strength is the primary goal of this system. One repetition with maximum resistance is performed. While keeping the resistance constant, single repetitions are executed and interspersed with a brief rest (fifteen to thirty seconds). This continues until the resistance can no longer be lifted, and at this point a new exercise is introduced.

(M) *Split Routine*—The individual trains from four to six days per week. On one day, the upper body is conditioned and on the following day—the lower body is involved. Some believe this system enables them to perform more work with less fatigue as they concentrate on specific parts of the body.

The selection of systems should be based upon predetermined goals. If muscular tone, endurance, and aerobic qualities are desired, either circuit training or the peripheral heart system are applicable. Pure muscular strength and mass are derived from the cheating technique and also using some form of heavy and light system.

Conclusive evidence demonstrating the advantages and disadvantages of one system over another does not exist. This area is fertile ground for research.

PROGRAM EXPERIENCE III

Example A—Weight Training Routine

Introductory routine—one set of from eight to ten repetitions for each exercise.

1. **'Swing'** (Warm-up for all Large Muscle Groups—Use minimal resistance)

Stand with feet spread to shoulder width. Hold a light dumbbell or plate overhead with arms extended. Begin exercise by bending knees and swinging resistance between legs. Return to the overhead position. Keep the elbows locked throughout the entire movement.

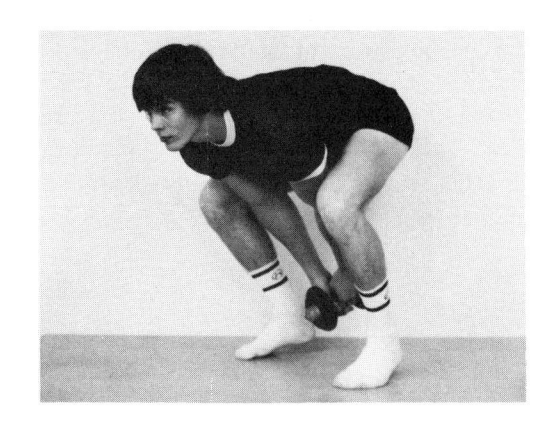

2. **'Clean and Press'** (Warm-up for all Large Muscle Groups—Use minimal resistance)

Stand with feet spread to shoulder width. Flex forward to waist—keeping knees locked and grasp the barbell with palms down and shoulder width grip. Raise weight to shoulder level with a vertical pulling motion while bending the elbows. Extend resistance to an overhead position being sure to lock the elbows. Reverse this movement to original position and repeat. The knees should be locked through the entire exercise.

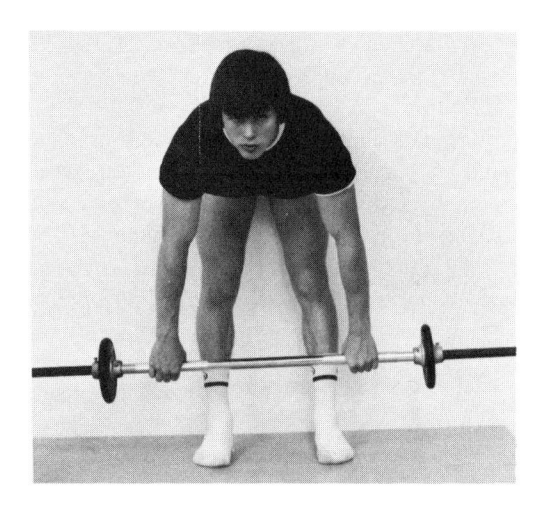

3. **'Good Morning'** (For Back and Hamstring)

Stand with feet spread to shoulder width. Hold a barbell behind the neck and resting on shoulders. Hand placement should be slightly wider than the shoulders. While keeping the knees locked, flex forward at the waist so that the upper body reaches a horizontal position, head in extended position. Reverse movement, extending up to a vertical position.

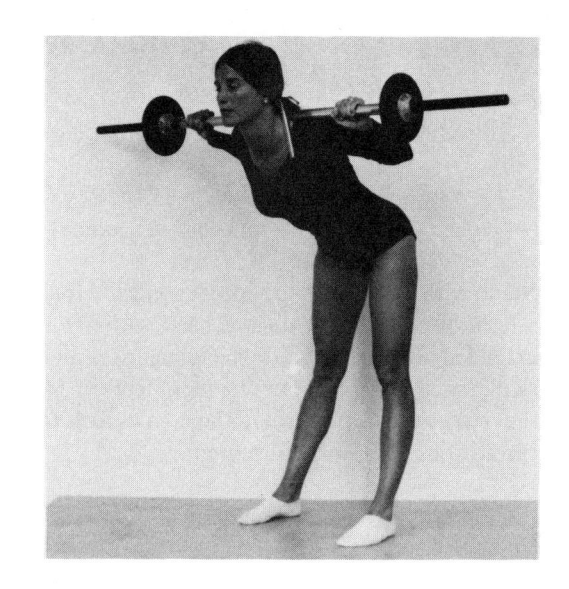

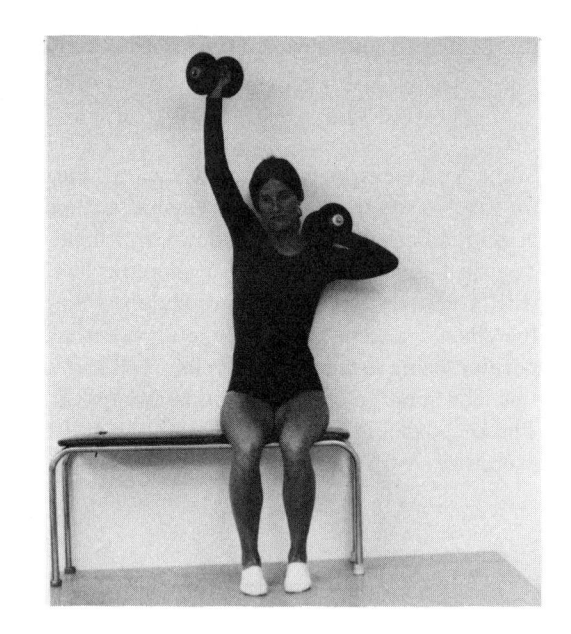

4. **'Dumbbell Alternate Press'** (Deltoid, Triceps and Upper Back)

Sitting position—hold a dumbbell in each hand in parallel position at shoulder level. Begin by extending one arm overhead and locking the elbow. Lower the resistance and at the same time extend the opposite arm overhead. Continue these alternating movements in rhythmic fashion.

5. **'Upright Rowing'** (Deltoid, Biceps, and Upper Back)

Stand with feet shoulder width apart. Hold a barbell in front of body—hands close together, palms down. Pull the resistance in a vertical direction to chin level, lower and repeat.

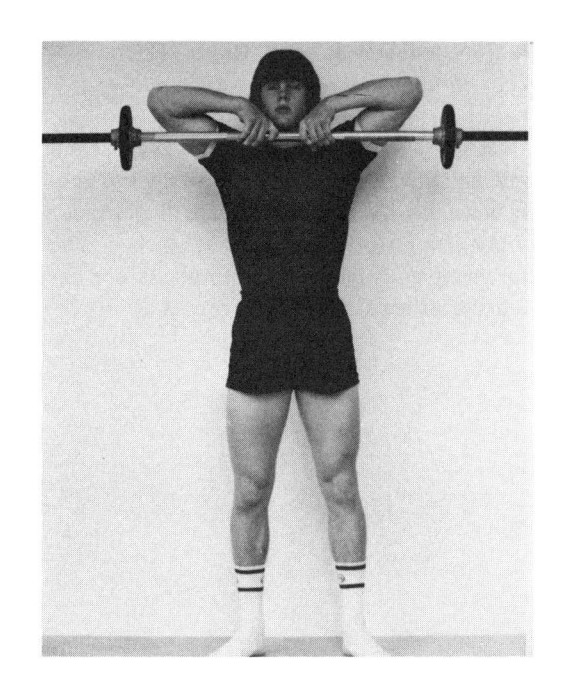

6. **'Military Press'** (Deltoid, Tricep, Upper Back)

Stand or sit with feet apart—grip the bar at shoulder width—palms down—clean the barbell to shoulder level. Extend the resistance to an overhead position and lock the elbows. Lower to shoulder level and repeat.

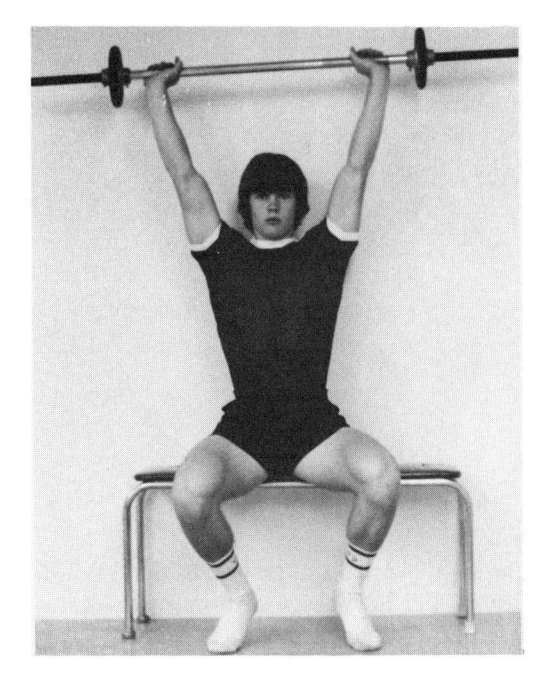

7. **'Dumbbell Lateral Raise'** (Deltoid—Trapezius)

Stand with feet apart. Hold dumbbells in each hand hanging at the side. With the palms facing down, lift the arms to the side in a circular motion being sure to keep elbows locked. The movement ends when the dumbbells are extended overhead. Lower and repeat.

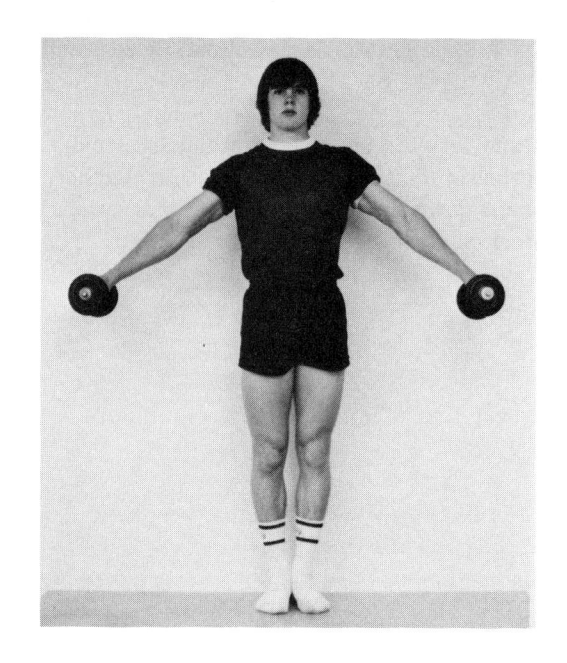

8. **'Leg Extensions'** (Quadriceps)

Sit with the lower legs hanging from the edge of a bench. While wearing weighted boots, extend the lower legs to a horizontal position, locking the knees. Lower and repeat.

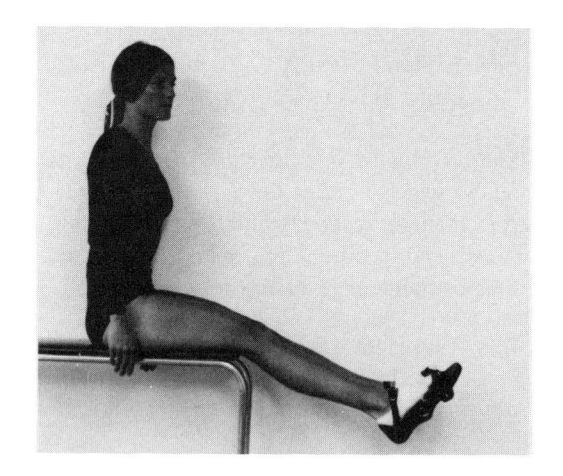

9. **'Leg Curl'** (Hamstring)

Lie on a bench in a prone position. While wearing weighted boots, curl the lower legs to a vertical position. Lower and repeat.

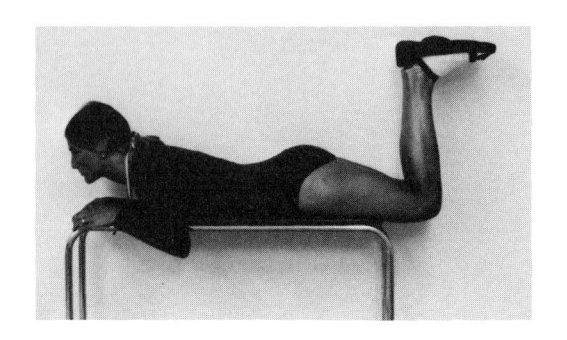

10. **'Toe Raise'** (Gastrocnemius)

Stand with feet six inches apart. Hold a barbell behind neck and resting on shoulders. Grip the barbell with the hands placed slightly wider than the shoulders. Raise body by extending toes. Lower and repeat. (Variations (1) toe in (2) toe out and (3) feet parallel.)

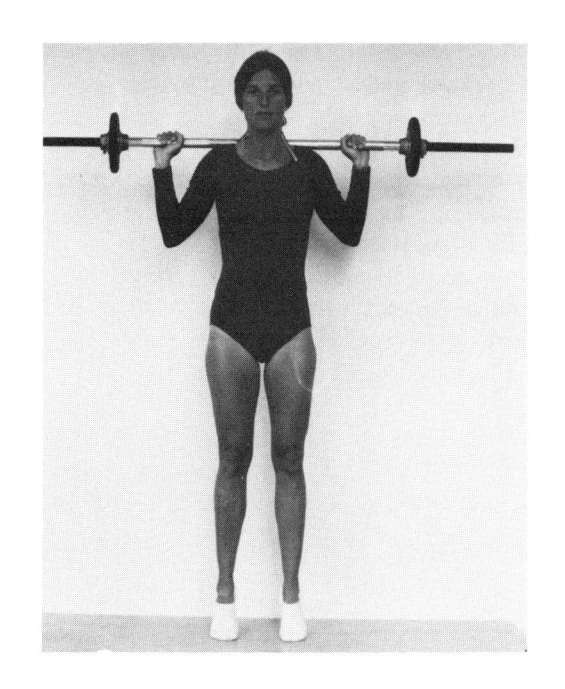

11. **'Deep Knee Bend'** (Hip and Knee Extensors)

Stand with feet spread at shoulder width. Hold a barbell behind the neck—resting on the upper back and shoulders. Grip the barbell slightly wider than shoulders. Bend the knees—lowering the body to a position in which the upper leg is parallel to the floor. Extend at the knees—moving back to a standing position and repeat. Keep back straight and head up during entire exercise.

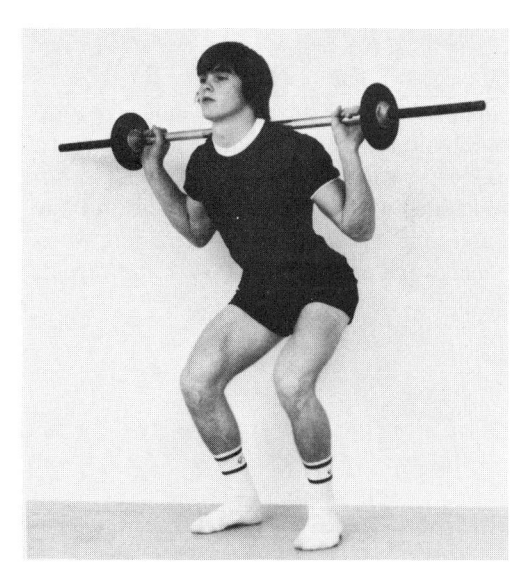

12. **'Dead Lift and Shoulder Shrug'** (Lower Back and Shoulder Girdle)

Stand with feet placed at shoulder width. Keep knees locked while flexing forward at the waist, grasp barbell with hands facing palms down at shoulder width. Raise upper body to a vertical position, keeping arms straight and continue movement by rotating shoulder forward, up and back. Lower and repeat.

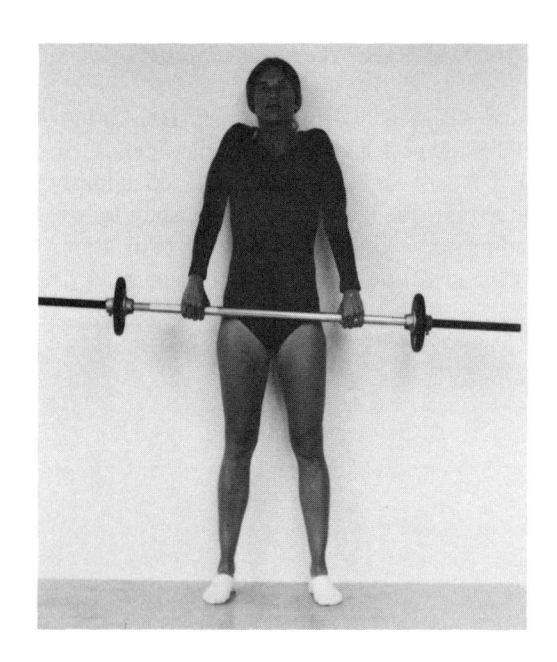

13. **'Bent Rowing'** (Upper Back—Latissimus—Biceps)

Stand with feet placed at shoulder width. While maintaining locked knees, bend forward and grasp barbell with the palms facing down at shoulder width. Flex elbows and pull the resistance in a vertical direction ending when it touches the upper chest. Lower and repeat.

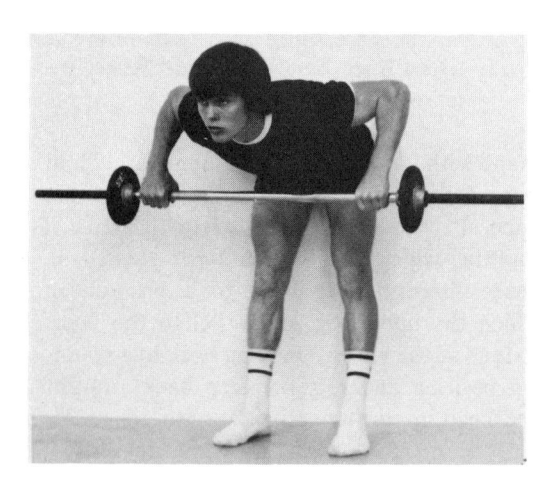

14. **'Curls'** (Biceps)

Stand with feet apart. Hold barbell hanging against the upper legs—with palms facing forward, arms extended, elbows at the side. Curl the barbell by flexing the lower arm and raise to shoulder level. Lower and repeat.

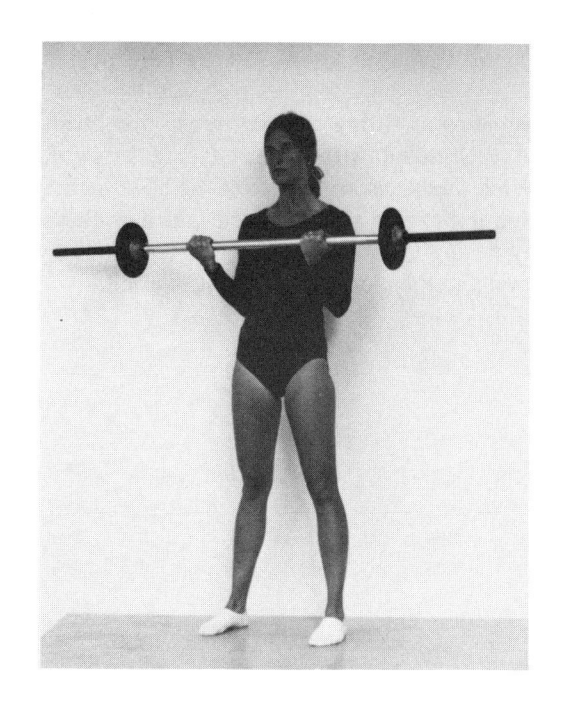

15. **'French Curl'** (triceps)

Stand or sit with feet apart. Hold a barbell behind head with palms facing up using narrow grip. Elbows facing forward, extend the upper arm so that the resistance will move in an arc and end in a vertical position. Lower and repeat.

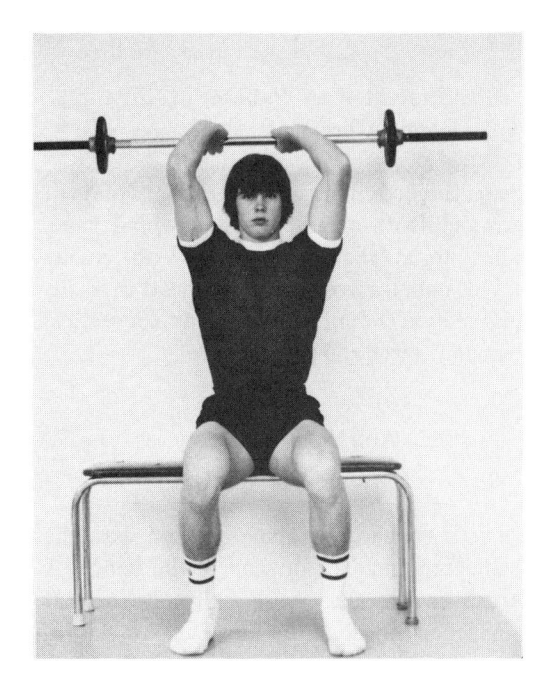

16. 'Dumbbell Alternate Curl' (Biceps)

Standing or sitting position, grasp dumbbells in each hand with palms facing forward. While the arms are extended—elbows at the side of the body, alternately curl the dumbbells by flexing the lower arm ending at shoulder level and then lower to original position.

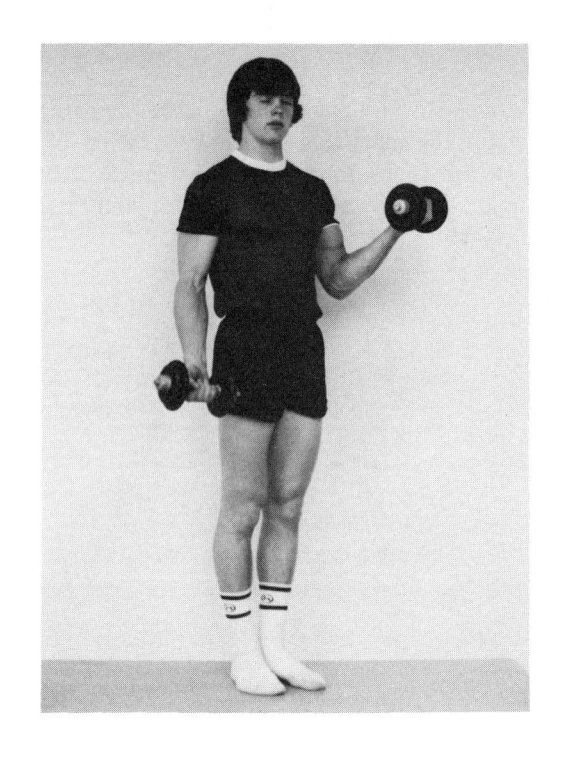

17. 'Straight Arm Pullover' (Latissimus-Dorsi—Chest)

Lie on the floor in a supine position. Hold the resistance with arms extended behind head, palms up at shoulder width. With elbows locked, pull the resistance overhead in a circular motion ending with the arms in a vertical position. Lower and repeat.

18. 'Bent Arm Pullover' (Pectorals—Latissimus)

Lie on a bench in a supine position with the head extending over the end of the bench. A barbell on the chest with palms up and at shoulder width. Push up and back so the resistance is extended and lowered past the head. The resistance will move in a circular motion. When the resistance reaches the floor, reverse the motion and repeat.

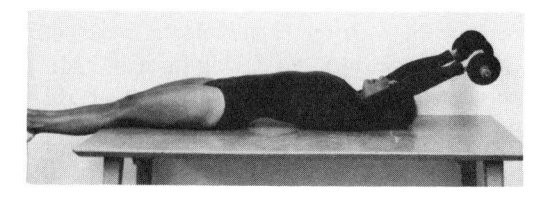

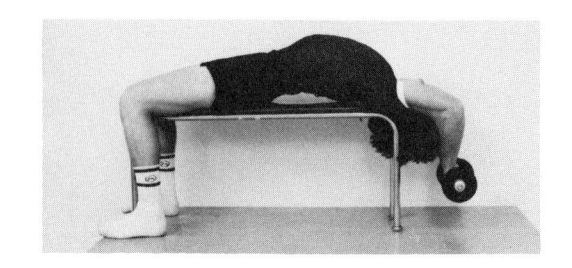

19. **'Dumbbell Cross'** (Pectorals—Biceps—Deltoids)

Lie on a bench in a supine position. Grasp a dumbbell in each hand. Support them in an overhead position with palms facing each other. Bend the elbows slightly and lower the dumbbells to the side. Stop just as the range of motion no longer permits movement. Reverse the circular motion and as the dumbbells reach an overhead position, allow them to pass each other creating extended movement. Reverse and repeat.

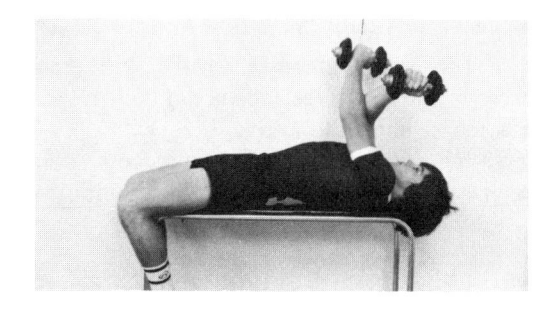

20. **'Bench Press'** (Triceps—Chest)

Lie in a supine position on a bench. Support a barbell on the chest, holding it with palms forward and at shoulder width. Raise the resistance in a vertical direction by extending the lower arms. Lock elbows, lower and repeat.

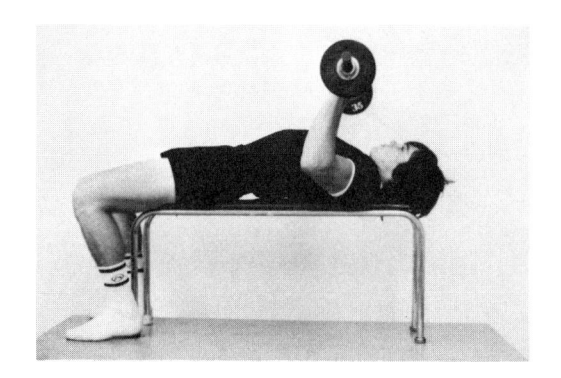

Example B—Body Resistance Routine

If weights are not readily available, the body can become a form of resistance. The following exercise routine suggests the use of body resistance as the catalyst for stimulating the development of strength and endurance.

Introductory routine—one set of from eight to ten repetitions for each exercise routine. Should be executed in quick, precise and rhythmical movements, utilizing the full-range of movement.

1. **'Jumping Jack'** (Total Body)

   a. Upright starting position—arms at side.
   b. On the count of one, jump to side stride, arms sideward and upward.
   c. Return to starting position on the count of two.

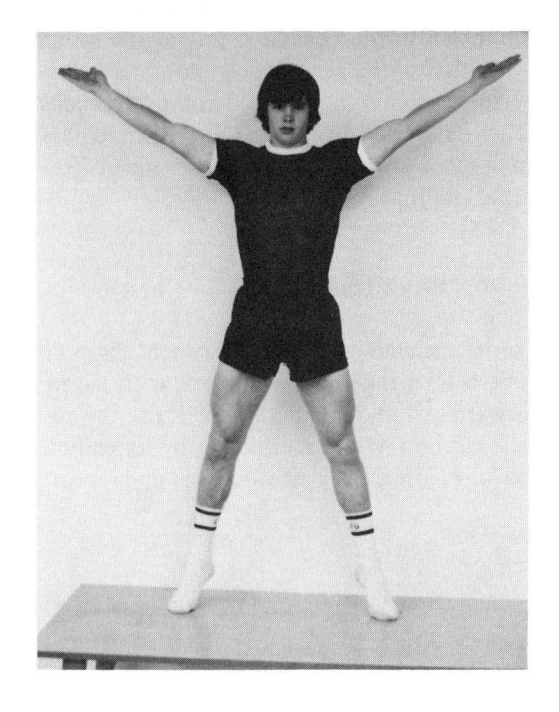

2. **'Arm Slinger'** (Pectorals—Shoulders)

a. Upright starting position—fists clenched, arms flexed at the elbow, arms parallel to ground.
b. Snap back arms at the shoulders for three counts.
c. On the count of four—open arms to the side—palms up.

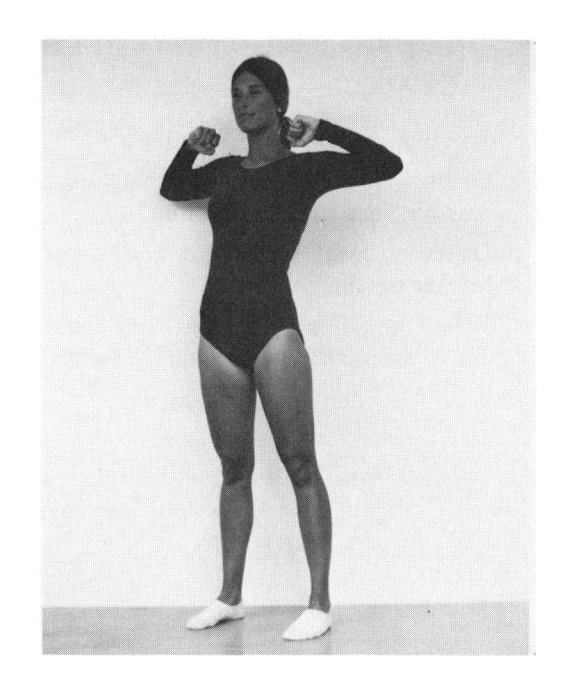

3. **'Alternate Toe Touch'** (Lower Back— External Obliques)

a. Standing position, feet apart, arms stretched to side.
b. On the first count—flex forward and sideward, touching the left toe with the right hand.
c. Return to the starting position on the count of two.
d. On the third count, alternate touching the right toe with the left hand.

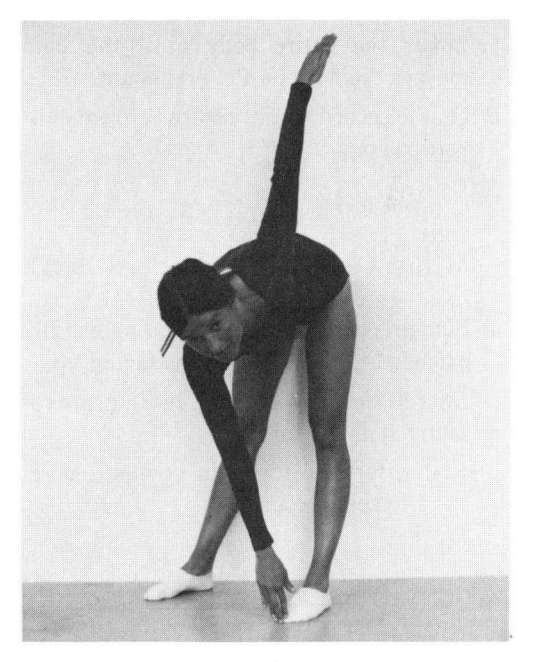

4. **'Deep Knee Bend'** (Hip and Knee Extensors)

a. Standing position—hands on hips.
b. On the first count, lower to a half squat position, back straight, head up.
c. On second count, squat lower until upper legs are parallel to floor.
d. Return to half squat on the third count and to the original position on the fourth.

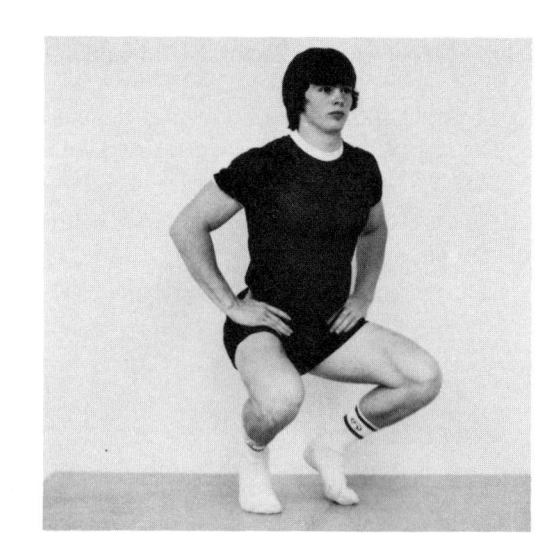

5. **'Push-ups'** (Triceps—Pectorals)

a. Front support position—body fully extended, hands shoulder width apart.
b. Lower the entire body until the chin touches the floor on the first count.
c. On the second count, return to front support position.

6. **'Arm Circles'** (Deltoid—Upper Back)

a. Standing position—arms and fingers fully extended to the side—palms facing up.
b. Inscribe circles with the fingers, arms rotating at the shoulder.
c. Rotate forward for eight counts and reverse for eight counts.

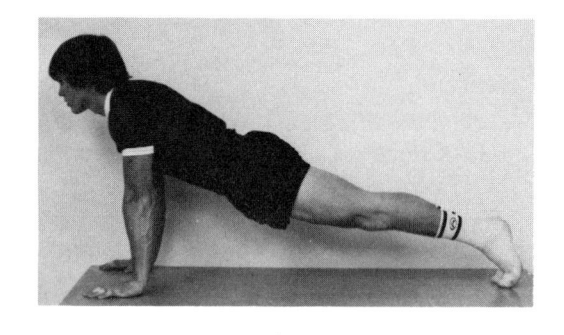

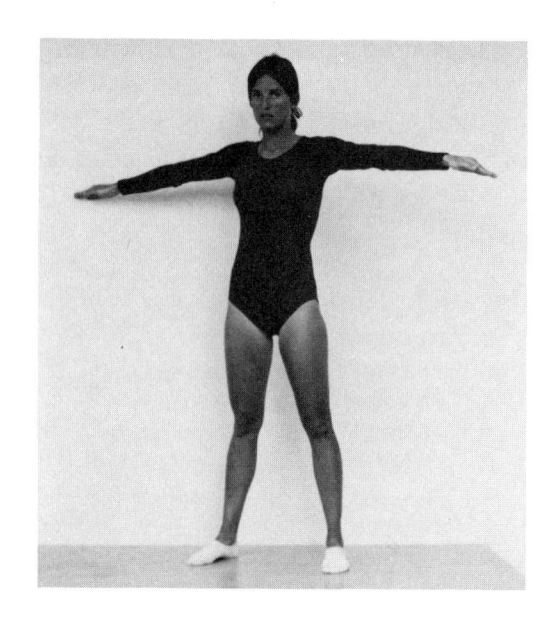

7. **'Sprinter'** (Total Body)

a. Front support position—draw the right knee up to the right elbow.
b. On the count of one, draw left knee up to left elbow as the right leg is extended back.
c. Alternate the legs on the second count.

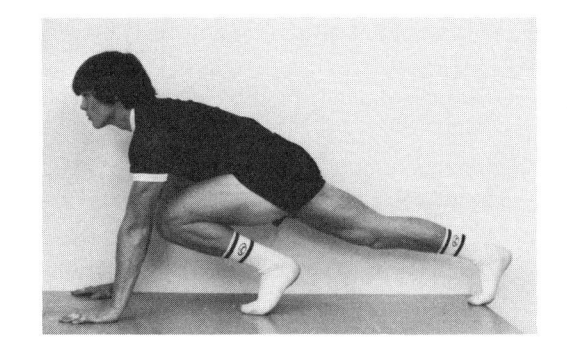

8. **'Curl-Up'** (Abdominals)

a. Supine starting position (on back)—interlock the fingers behind the neck—draw feet up to buttocks—knees apart.
b. On the count of one, roll body upward—attempt to touch elbows to floor—arms inside of knees.
c. Return to starting position on the count of two.

9. **'Tuck Sit-ups'** (Abdominal—Hip Flexors)

a. Supine starting position—body fully extended with arms overhead.
b. At the first count, raise the upper body as the legs are brought up to the tuck position. Reach outside the knees with the arms.
c. On the second count, return to starting position.

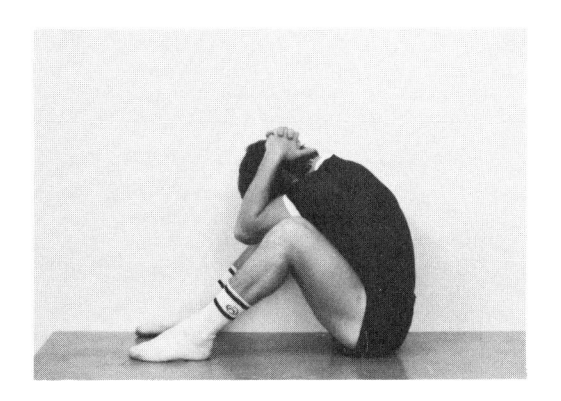

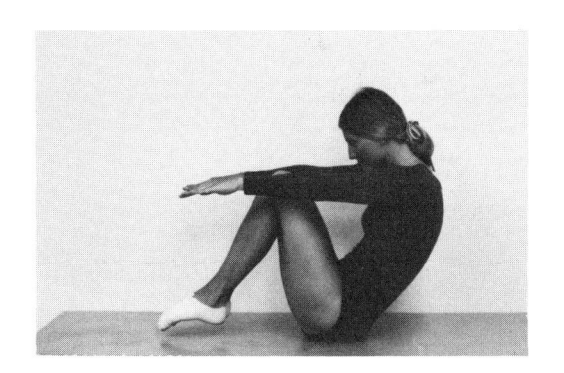

10. **'Squat Extensions'** (Total Body)

a. Upright starting position—hands to the side.
b. On the first count, execute deep knee bend—placing hands on the floor—between the knees.
c. On the second count, extend the body to a front support position.
d. Return to squat position on the count of three.
e. On fourth count, return to starting position.

11. **'Swimmer'** (Shoulder—Back and Buttocks)

a. Prone starting position—arms, body and legs fully extended.
b. Raise the upper and lower body by creating an arch in the lower back.
c. Holding the arms extended—alternate moving them up and down.
d. Simultaneously—with the legs extended—toes pointed back—flutter kick from the hips.

12. **'Sprint and Jog'** (Hips and Legs)

a. Upright starting position—arms slightly flexed at the side.
b. Jog in place—raise the knees for sixteen counts.
c. Sprint for sixteen counts.
d. Alternate jogging and sprinting.

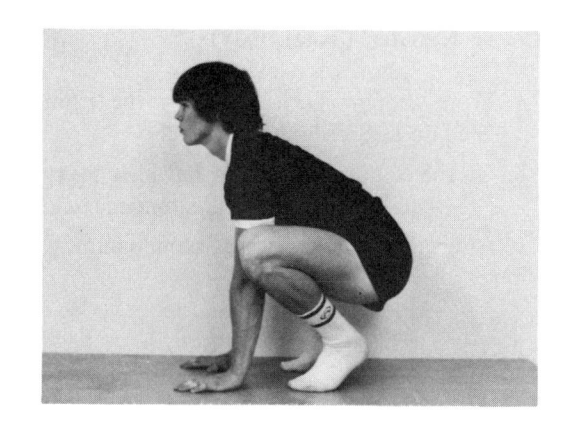

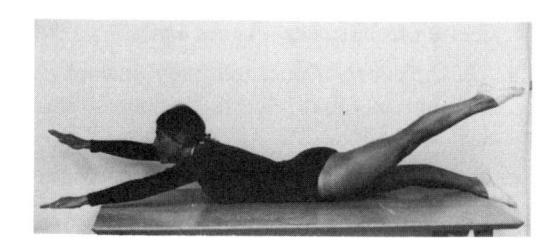

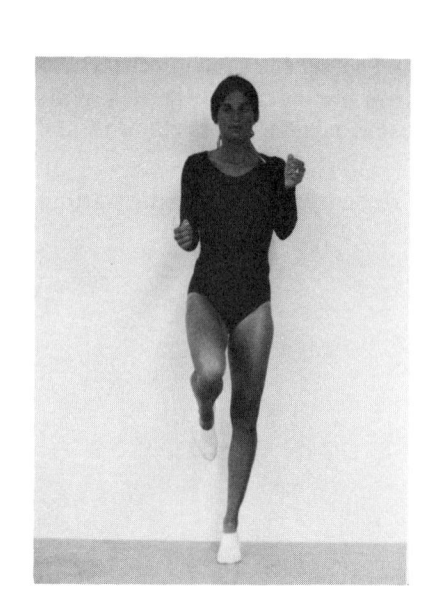

EIGHTEEN MINUTE WONDER WORKOUT

We offer the "eighteen minute wonder workout" as a practical, efficient and vigorous means of achieving high levels of conditioning. The training regimen should be initiated in stages. The program elicits training increases in all of the primary components. The following directions and procedures will provide all the information which is necessary to experience the wonder workout.

1. In starting, reduce the times and suggested repetitions for each phase of the workout by 50 percent.
2. For the first three training periods, expend minimal effort in performing each of the activities. Gradually increase your intensity as your body starts realizing training effects.
3. When you reach the stage of expending near maximum effort for the entire nine minutes, gradually increase the time and number of repetitions in each of the activities until finally reaching the recommended limits.
4. The entire training program can be accomplished in a small room by substituting running in place rather than using the track.
5. If you reach conditioning levels that permit you to persist with high intensity for eighteen minutes, you can increase the level of activity by:
   a. adding repetitions.
   b. increasing the time limit for each activity.
   c. increasing the resistance at each progressive resistance station.
   d. decreasing the time of completing the progressive resistance circuit.
   e. increasing the intensity of effort while running and performing abdominal exercise.
   f. performing additional progressive resistance mini-circuits or trying two wonder workouts.
6. The wonder workout is designed as a large circuit in which the individual moves from one station to the next without resting.
7. If a multistationed progressive machine is available, have the resistance correctly loaded before beginning the workout.
8. If a large group of individuals is exercising at one time, arrange two groups so that one group is running while the other is utilizing progressive resistance exercises, followed by abdominal work. Change stations after nine minutes.
9. Utilize a rhythmic cadence during abdominal and resistance exercise.
10. Use a clock or stopwatch to measure the elapsed time at each station.

18-Minute Wonder Workout

No.	Repetitions	Lbs. Resistance	Time	Activity	Exercise
1				Stretching	
			10 sec.		Hurdler Rt. Front
			10 sec.		Hurdler Rt. Back
			10 sec.		Hurdler Lt. Front
			10 sec.		Hurdler Lt. Back
2				Running	
			8 min.		In Place, Track, Field, Street
3				Abdominal	
	20		40 sec.		Leg Raise
	25		40 sec.		Curl Ups (knees up and to the side)
	50		70 sec.		Half Sits (fast pace)
4				Progressive Resistance	
	12		40 sec.		Toe Raise
	12		40 sec.		Bench Press
	12		40 sec.		Reverse Curl
	12		40 sec.		Leg Curl
	12		40 sec.		Upright Rowing
	12		40 sec.		Press
	12		40 sec.		Dumbbell Curl
	12		40 sec.		Bent Rowing
	12		40 sec.		Leg Press
	12		40 sec.		French Curl
	12		40 sec.		Latissimus Dorsi Pull
	12		40 sec.		Dips
5				Stretching	
			10 sec.		Taylor Sit
			10 sec.		Good Morning

Selected References

Asmussen, E. Growth in muscular strength and power in L. Paric (Ed.) Physical activity: Human Growth and Development. New York: Academic Press, 1973.

Brown, C. H., and Wilmore J. H. The effects of maximal resistance training on the strength and body composition of women athletes. *Medicine and Science in Sports,* 1974, 6, 174–177.

Hislop, H. J., Perrine, J. J. The isokenetic concept of exercise, *Physical Therapy,* 1967, 47, 114–117.

Wilmore, J. H. Weight training for women, *Fitness for Living,* 1973, Nov./Dec., 40–45.

Withers, R.: Effect of varied weight-training loads on the strength of university freshman. *Research Quarterly:* 41: 110–114, 1970.

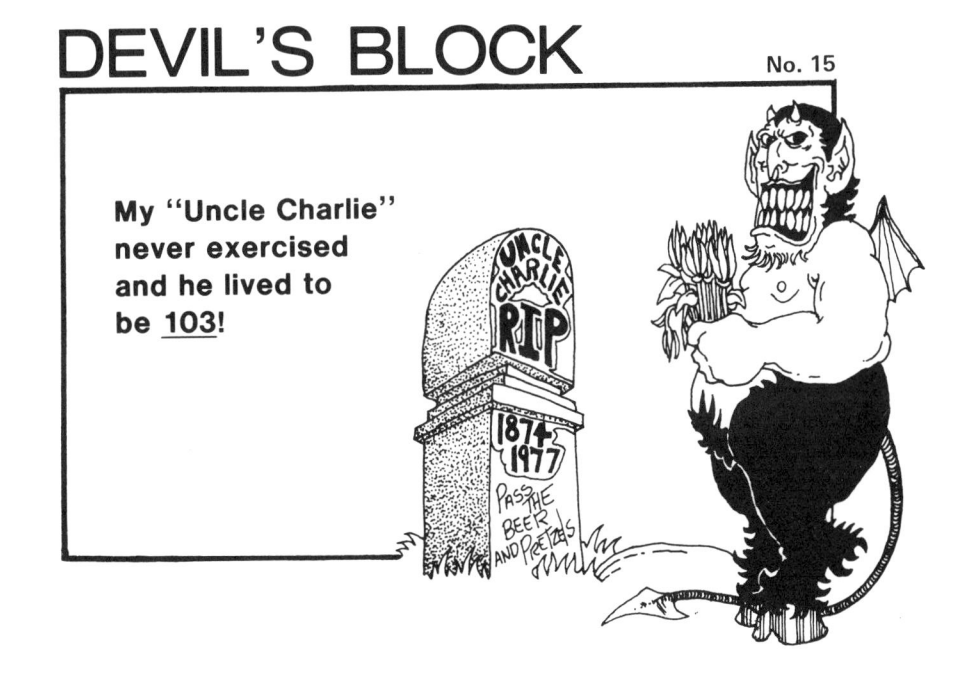

DEVIL'S BLOCK   No. 15

My "Uncle Charlie" never exercised and he lived to be 103!

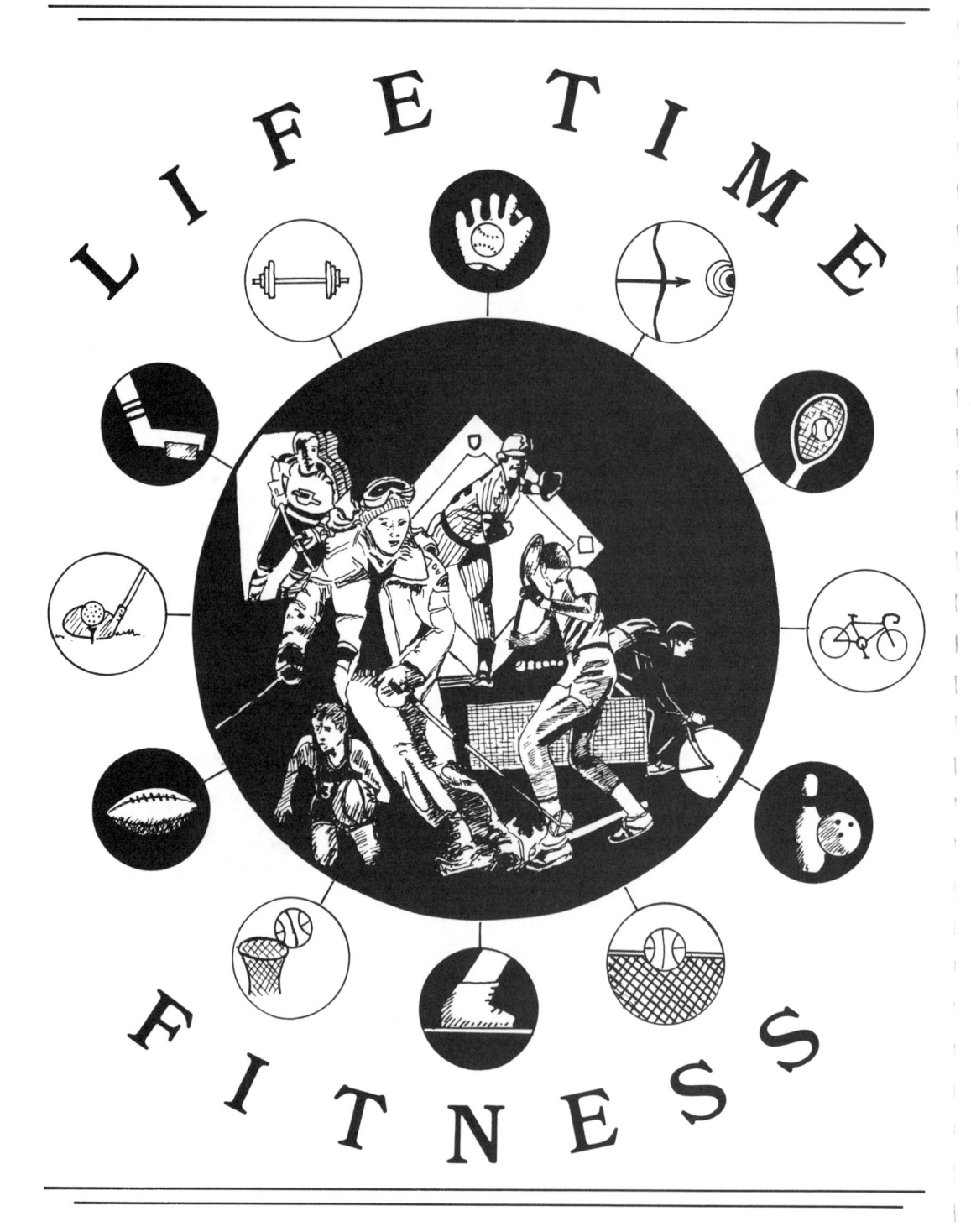

SECTION III—SPECTRUM OF SPORTS ACTIVITIES

LIFE TIME FITNESS

Section III
SPECTRUM OF SPORTS ACTIVITIES

Sport is a dominating form of expression in Physical Exercise and all forms of active leisure pursuits. Sport signifies the striving to succeed in physical efficiency, through the acquisition of skills and the application of strategies in contests.

This section introduces the broad spectrum of sport activities. A natural outgrowth of gaining skills in sports is the desire to test these skills in competitive challenges. Conversely, competitive challenges provide incentive for the development of physical skills. For this reason, the merits of entering the competitive arena should be considered.

The spectrum of sports is divided into three classifications; (1) individual, (2) small groups, and (3) large groups. Classifying sports in this manner, rather than child, teenage, adult or lifetime activities, establishes patterns that may be followed or developed whenever and wherever the environment permits, the participants are available and/or the inclination is present. In addition, the underlying selection for any activity should be pleasure and health related benefits.

Many sports are seasonal in nature. Although most indoor sports (basketball, handball, badminton) can be played year round, many outdoor sports are of limited duration because of climatic conditions (snow skiing, softball, and water skiing). Other sports such as swimming and tennis can be engaged in either environment. We would encourage individuals to engage in several sports each year, each in its own season. This scheme would tend to preserve a zest for each sport.

In addition, participation in a variety of sports assists in the development and maintenance of the primary and motor performance components of fitness.

The section is concluded with Personal Appraisal No. 14, "The Individualized Activity Program." Through use of this appraisal, we wish each of you to be the inventor of a personalized program of activity. Your specific needs will be the primary factor in the selection, organization and execution of the program.

16
INTRODUCTION TO COMPETITION

Sections I and II have provided a foundation of principles and concepts regarding the reaction of the human body to programs of physical activity. This section introduces the exciting, wide, wonderful world of sport.

As you enter this arena, we would like you to accept the following challenges:

1. Select a variety of sports which appeal to you.
2. Show the pioneer spirit and have the courage to enter new domains. There is excitement in learning new skills.
3. On rare occasions, one can learn to improve skill in the role of a spectator, but for the most part be an active participant! This will help to maintain and improve your level of fitness.
4. Experience the true satisfaction of perfecting skill. Many of us merely scratch the surface in reaching our true potential. *Action* speaks louder than words! One speaks of wanting to excel, to become outstanding, but if he does not practice, train or watch his diet . . . in reality, *he does not want to excel*!
5. Learn to cope with the stress in competitive situations with poise and confidence. Sports participation becomes an emotionally healthy and exciting adventure if you have the temperament to test your skill level against the skills of others.

Competitive Arena

"The fun of competition is in striving to win." We submit that enjoyment, competition and winning are compatible. This constitutes the competitive arena. In competition, winners are those who strive to do their best. The pleasure and satisfaction derived from the competition results when this principle is in effect. The true "winner" is one who can leave the competitive endeavor with the knowledge that regardless of the final score, he has exerted his best effort.

Value of Competition

When "competition" becomes the topic of a conversation, some people immediately withdraw for they perceive the term to imply solely winning or losing. Winning involves the spirit of competition. It has always been an immediate objective in sport, but it cannot be an end in itself.

Competition must be put within a framework in which winning is characterized by positive forms of behavior. When conducted with integrity, sport and competition can be a guiding force in preparing all of us for an enriching and vital role in life.

There are varied viewpoints as to the value of competition. Remarks to the effect that competition is dehumanizing and develops undue aggressiveness have been noted. Some former athletes have displayed their disdain for competition often in severe, sensationalized terms. Their philosophies may reflect the negative aspects of winning at any cost. Their criticisms, we feel, do not represent the true spirit and conduct of the vast number of dedicated individuals in the competitive arena.

While it is true that negative effects can emerge, they may well be due to a superimposed outside influence that seeks some personal gain from turmoil. Most sociologists and psychologists view sports and competition as healthy pursuits for most individuals. The competition arena, when not subjected to manipulation by a few, provides a laboratory for the expression of individual and group skills. Moreover, the competitor learns the vast difference between performing in a virtual vacuum and performing under the stress of competition.

The manner in which competitiveness is instilled in athletics is of extreme importance. We submit, competition can be positive or negative, depending upon the method in which it is conducted. Since sport and competition are expanding at a rapid rate, e.g., tennis, soccer and wrestling; it seems obvious that people are seeking that challenge. We must learn how to compete. We should have a strong desire to win, but within the framework of the established rule. You *win—through development of skill and giving every bit you have in your performance.* As soon as competition leaves this framework, it can become a negative experience.

The Framework for Healthy Competition

1. We should compete—we should strive to win—with honesty and compassion.
2. The won-lost record cannot be an end in itself.
3. Leadership should reflect concern for team members and personal integrity.
4. Will to win can be used as a motivating force in learning.
5. The competitive arena should not be dictated to from the whims of spectators who view each contest with vested interests.

Learning Environment

Involvement in a competitive situation can be a great learning experience. We believe that many lessons in life become more meaningful as a result of participation on the playing fields where competition prevails.

A major role of education is to create situations in which students will develop an understanding and respect for other people. It does not take long to discern the nature of self, teammates and opponents in competitive situations. Truth is something we cherish as a quality of civilized life. In the quest of truth, we must first know ourselves. To know self, what better way than to be placed in a competitive situation in which the will to win prevails and in which stress and conflict may occur. Competition in sport activities necessitates emotional control. How we react to the challenge of stress and conflict is an indication of our personality and character.

In this situation, the reactions of the participants become revealing:

1. Are rules circumvented in pursuit of victory?
2. Are others belittled to cover mistakes?
3. Are officials chastised?
4. Are lame excuses invented to hide inadequacies?
5. Is the intent of participation self-grandiosement?

These are some negative patterns which can occur throughout life in stress situations. Face life more realistically and honestly as exemplified by the following concepts:

1. There can be no satisfaction in a dishonest victory.
2. Blaming and chastising others for one's own incompetency is an indication of a personality weakness.
3. Each individual must decide the relative importance of excellence. Excellence can only be achieved through improved proficiency. Therefore, there must be a willingness to take the necessary steps to improve skills.

As we gain experience in the competitive arena, self-evaluation becomes a very important tool in the decision making process. For example if a loss occurs, we can make a realistic evaluation of the factors which contributed to the loss. If logic prevails, an important decision must be made. What skills can I improve upon so that future challenges lead to different results?

First Decision—If your decision is to achieve greater excellence, it becomes a simple matter to go back to the practice courts, fields or swimming pool where constant practice and intense effort will improve your weaknesses so that you will be better prepared to overcome adversity.

Second Decision—If, in light of your competitive experience, you place less value on achieving a high skill level and exposure to intense competition, this type of stress is not for you! The most important follow-up action to this second decision is to remain physically active and at the level of competition which is pleasurable so that you will:

1. Better understand yourself
2. Learn about others
3. Find out how you and others react to challenge
4. Know how to cope with stress
5. Experience winning in striving to do your best

A form of competition has prevailed through Section I and Section II. You have followed a pattern of self-competition during the "Personal Appraisals" while participating in the "program experiences." Improvement in one's self is a form of competition since we compete against our previous standards.

Summary

We feel that for most people the environment of competitive sport is ideal. Within this framework stress may occur. Athletes must continually prove themselves. On the basketball court, badminton court, in the swimming pool or on the football field, the athlete is constantly challenged. The competitive situation can become a negative experience if the athlete becomes complacent or cannot cope with stress.

As individuals are exposed to competition, they should ascertain their levels of achievement in order to make objective decisions. They have to decide that they are willing to serve their apprenticeship to achieve a higher level of skill. There are some who are unwilling to expend the time and effort required for a championship performance and place their values elsewhere. They have acquired knowledge of self and understand their strengths and weaknesses. They are now better able to make personal adjustments in life.

Interaction between and among participants in an athletic contest often becomes one of those beautiful moments in interpersonal relations. We admit that, at times, behavior in the name of competition results in negative or uncomplimentary exchanges. The incidents, we trust, will remain rare. Let us consider, instead, the great realm of appreciation, the exhilaration or the lasting stimulation from scoring a goal against all odds; or observing your opponent moving through time and space in a graceful effort to return your best shot; or the great pleasure aroused by a team effort to accomplish the physically uncommon feat. These are some of the concomitant joys of competitive sports.

Selected References

Braver, S. Reciprocity, Cohesiveness and cooperation in two person games. *Psychological Reports,* 1975, 36, 371–378.

Coplin, T. H. Isometric Exercise; clinical usage. *Journal of Athletic Trainers Association,* 1971, 6, 110–114.

Coplin, T. H. Isometric Exercise; clinical usage. *Journal of National Athletic Trainers Association,* 1971, 6, 110–114.

Costill, D. L. Effects of physical training in men with coronary heart disease. *Medicine and Science in Sports,* 1974, 6 (2), 95.

Edwards, H. Sociology of sport. Homewood, Ill.: Dorsey Press, 1973.

Ellis, M. G. Why people play. Englewood Cliffs, N.J.: Prentice-Hall, 1973.

Spreitzer, E., Pugh, M. Interscholastic athletics and educational aspirations. *Sociology of Education,* 1973, 46, 171–182.

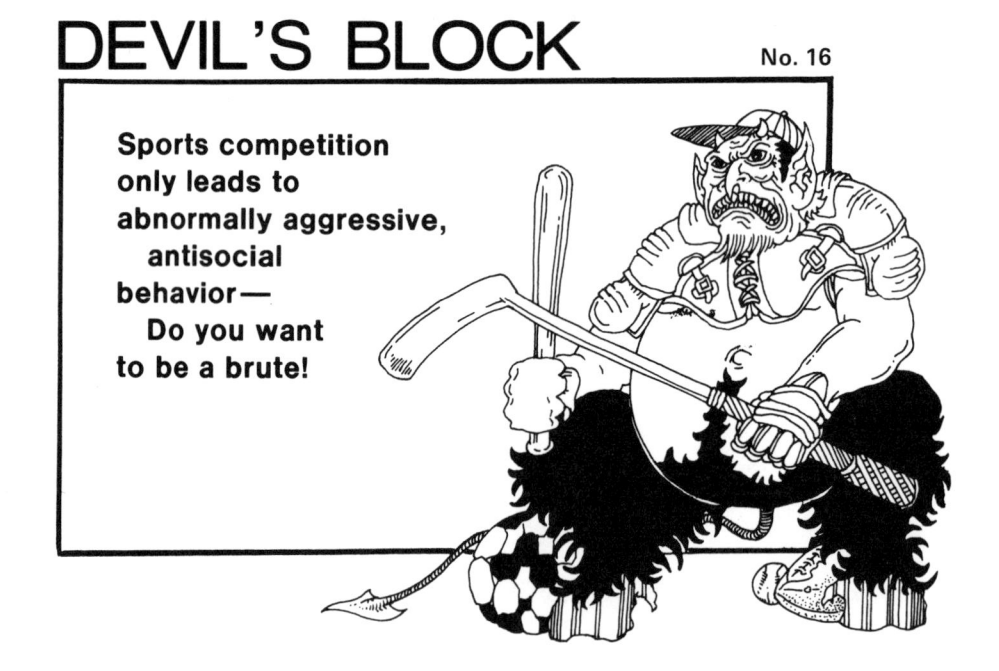

DEVIL'S BLOCK   No. 16

**Sports competition only leads to abnormally aggressive, antisocial behavior—
Do you want to be a brute!**

17
ANALYSIS OF THE SPORT ACTIVITIES

The broad spectrum of sport activities available to us offers a multitude of pleasurable experiences and health-related values. Some forms of play are prohibitive in that an abundance of time may be required and specific climates and geography may be necessitated. Unfortunately, these limitations remove enticing opportunities for pleasurable activity from many individuals. However, most sport forms (i.e., dance, bowling and table tennis) are within the reach of the majority of our population. In recent years, a number of recreation palaces have been constructed in which year-round participation in skating, tennis, handball, squash, swimming, weight training, self-defense, etc., are offered. As leisure time becomes more prevalent, this trend might well become the wave of the future.

Individuals confronted with physical limitations and disabilities need not be discouraged from participation since there is a great variety of activity from which to choose. Most sport forms can be adapted to accommodate the handicapped, as in the case of wheelchair basketball. Some severely disabled people have had success while participating in major sport competition. There have been blind wrestlers, skiers and golfers. We often find a football player, swimmer, or skier who becomes so highly motivated by a sport that he overcomes a handicap sometimes severe enough to inhibit most of us. Heart patients often find that walking and jogging are recommended forms of therapy. Virtually all people, regardless of what their handicap may be, can realize success and enjoyment from sport.

Our purpose in presenting this chapter is to analyze the means through which sport activities can assist, and in some cases, replace the core activities in bringing forth health-related training effects. Virtually all of the activities discussed offer excellent opportunities for emotional release and stress adaptation. Through a careful analysis of the sport forms which provoke our interests, we are better able to design logical and effective lifetime activity programs.

The broad spectrum of activities are organized into three categories: individual, small group and large group activities. Our purpose in structuring the spectrum in this manner is two-fold. First, we offer a system of classification which encourages a selection of activity for those individuals who continually shun sports because they are unable to find others with similar interests. Second, we differentiate between sports in which individual effort may be the determining factor in successful accomplishment and sports requiring the blending of individual talent with others through cooperation and advanced team strategy for successful performance.

Individual Sport Activities

1. Archery
2. Bowling
3. Canoeing
4. Cross Country
5. Diving
6. Golf
7. Horseback Riding
8. Horseshoes
9. Scuba Diving
10. Skiing
11. Trampoline
12. Tumbling

Although individual sport activities may involve opponents and team scoring, they are also characterized by the ability of a person to realize successful physical performance even without opponents or teammates. When placed in the competitive situation, individuals must rely on their own abilities while seeking the heights of performance. They must be able to summon reserves of strength, courage and stress tolerance. The pursuit of excellence in individual activities can be lonely, requiring strength of personality and character.

The activities listed vary greatly in their ability to elicit training effects. Sports such as bowling, horseshoes and archery are virtually incapable of producing training effects in the primary components of conditioning. Conversely, canoeing, skiing and trampolining can yield aerobic-anaerobic benefits and strength increases of high quality. Explosive power and speed are unaffected by bowling and horseshoes. However, these same qualities are influenced through participation in cross country and tumbling. The following principle holds true for virtually all sport activities:

As movement, coordination, and change of direction requirements increase, the potential for efficient motor performance abilities is increased.

The individual sport activities are capable of providing emotional release and relief from tension and stress. These forms of play are often conducted out-of-doors, bringing the participants in touch with nature. This can have a valuable spiritual effect on many people.

Each individual activity can be adapted or adjusted to bring forth additional training effects. An increased pace while playing golf or even jogging the fairways would raise the heart rate to levels in which cardio-respiratory benefits will result. In archery, use of heavier poundage bows will promote shoulder and upper back strength. Combining the juggling of balls and bouncing on the trampoline will result in heightened eye-hand coordination. With imagination, all forms of sport can be altered to provide additional conditioning benefits.

Small Group Activities

1. Badminton
2. Dance (Folk, Square, Social)
3. Handball
4. Racquetball
5. Rhythmic Gymnastics
6. Self-Defense
7. Squash
8. Table Tennis
9. Tennis
10. Wrestling

Small group activities usually require from two to four participants. An important factor limiting potential improvement in virtually all sport activities is the relative competence of the opponent. As the quality of performance and intensity of effort of the opponent decreases, so does the probability of self-improvement. As a general rule, participating with accomplished opponents may result in more efficient development of skills and conditioning.

Small group activities are capable of stimulating higher levels of motor performance benefits than most individual activities. The majority of group activities involve a variety of skills which continually require finite adjustments. This results in heightened skill levels and motor performance development.

Most of these activities, with the exception of wrestling, have a negligible influence on muscular strength. Some sport forms may promote muscular endurance in specific muscle groups. Small group activities can have a positive effect on cardio-respiratory function. However, the fact that each sport is interspersed with slight rest periods, i.e.; alternating of serve, halftime, changing of side; allows the heart brief recovery periods which limit aerobic benefits.

The small group activities offer relatively inexpensive opportunities for pleasurable forms of competition in which skill levels, primary components, and motor performance qualities, can be enhanced.

Large Group Activities

1. Basketball
2. Football (Touch)
3. Hockey (Field)
4. Lacrosse
5. Rugby
6. Soccer
7. Softball
8. Speedball
9. Volleyball
10. Waterpolo

Large group activities differ from individual and small group activities in the following manner. First, they utilize more contestants which adds to the complexity of sport and introduces the factor of group dynamics. The ebb and flow of participation are altered according to the state of psychological motivation of the group. Group membership and peer acceptance are outgrowths of participation.

Second, it is interesting to note that each of the large group activities requires intricate passing and catching skills. These skills involve timing, cooperation with others, and can be considered a foundation for team play.

Finally, the large group activities are team-oriented necessitating a mesh of individual personalities, attitudes and skills. The success of the team is dependent upon tlhe interplay, cooperation and unity of its members.

These sports are capable of stimulating a wide variety of conditioning benefits. They are similar to the small group activities in that brief rest periods are interspersed between bursts of maximal effort. They can promote aerobic benefits, but like the small group, they are inferior to the core activities in eliciting intense cardio-respiratory and muscular strength training effects. These sports produce increased skill levels and have a positive effect on the motor performance abilities.

The following chart provides a more explicit description of each activity comprising the spectrum of sport. It can be of great value in designing a personal lifetime program.

DEVIL'S BLOCK

No. 17

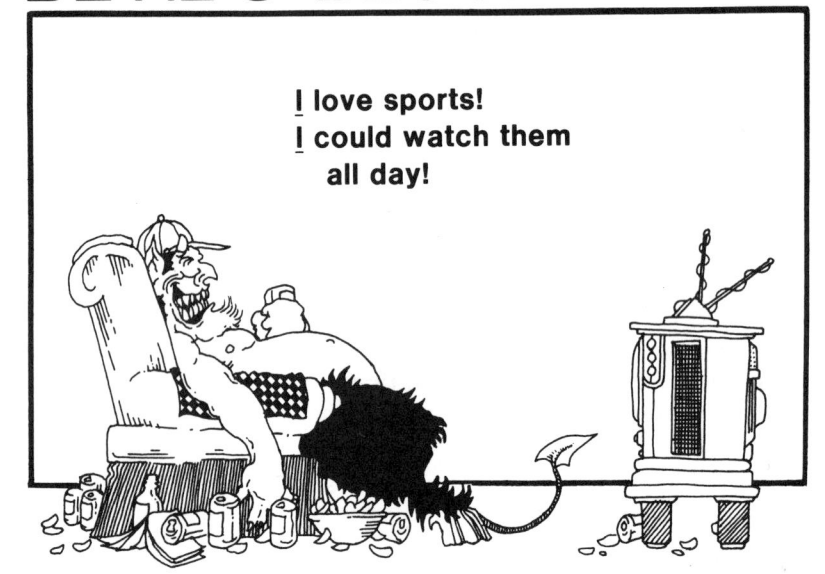

I love sports!
I could watch them
all day!

INTERPRETATION
Sports Activities Analysis Chart

This chart offers a comprehensive analysis of thirty-two activities that comprise the spectrum of sports. They are examined in terms of their potential for eliciting training benefits. The numerical symbol relating relative value is based upon our feelings of the extent of gain that can be expected as the average person expends time and effort. The exceptional individual able to tolerate high levels of stress may expect increased benefits of a higher level than those provided. The numerical values of the rating scale may change if the normal conduct of the sport is adapted or altered.

Sport Activities

Contribution to Components of Conditioning

Rating Scale
6 — Maximum Value
5 — Intense Value
4 — High Value
3 — Medium Value
2 — Low Value
1 — Minimal Value
0 — Zero Value

Sport Activities—Analysis Chart

Components of Conditioning	Body Symmetry	Cardio-Respiratory	Flexibility	Muscular Strength	Muscular Endurance	Speed	Coordination	Agility	Balance	Explosive Power	Posture	Weight Control	Total	Overall Average to Total Fitness
	II	III	IV	V	VI	VII	VIII	IX	X	XI	XII	XIII		
Individual Activities														
1. Archery	1	0	2	1	1	0	3	0	2	0	5	0	15	1.25
2. Bowling	0	0	1	1	1	0	3	2	2	0	2	0	12	1.00
3. Canoeing	4	5	2	4	5	1	3	2	4	3	3	4	40	3.33
4. Cross Country	4	6	3	2	4	5	3	3	3	3	4	6	46	3.83
5. Diving	2	2	5	2	2	1	5	4	5	4	5	2	38	3.17
6. Golf	1	1	3	0	2	0	4	1	3	2	3	1	21	1.75
7. Horseback Riding	0	3	1	1	2	0	3	0	3	0	3	1	17	1.41
8. Horseshoes	0	0	1	0	1	0	3	0	2	0	1	0	8	.67
9. Scuba-Diving	3	3	2	2	4	2	3	0	2	1	2	3	27	2.25
10. Downhill Skiing	3	3	2	2	3	3	5	3	6	2	3	3	38	3.17
11. Trampoline	4	3	4	3	4	1	5	4	5	3	2	3	41	3.42
12. Tumbling	4	2	5	3	4	2	5	4	5	5	4	3	46	3.83
Small Group Activities														
1. Badminton	2	3	3	1	2	3	4	3	3	3	2	3	32	2.67
2. Dance (Folk Square Social)	1	2	2	0	1	1	3	3	3	1	3	2	22	1.83
3. Handball	3	3	2	1	4	3	4	3	2	3	1	3	32	2.67
4. Racquetball	2	3	2	1	3	2	3	3	2	2	1	3	27	2.25
5. Rhythmic-Gymnastics	4	3	4	1	2	1	4	3	4	2	5	4	37	3.08
6. Self-Defense	3	2	4	2	2	3	2	3	3	3	3	2	32	2.67
7. Squash	2	3	2	1	3	2	3	4	3	1	2	3	29	2.42

Sport Activities—Analysis Chart, Continued

Components of Conditioning	Body Symmetry II	Cardio-Respiratory III	Flexibility IV	Muscular Strength V	Muscular Endurance VI	Speed VII	Coordination VIII	Agility IX	Balance X	Explosive Power XI	Posture XII	Weight Control XIII	Total	Overall Average to Total Fitness
8. Table Tennis	1	2	1	1	2	2	3	3	2	1	2	1	21	1.75
9. Tennis	3	3	2	1	3	3	3	3	2	1	2	3	29	2.42
10. Wrestling	5	4	5	4	6	2	3	4	3	5	1	4	46	3.83
Large Group Activities														
1. Basketball	2	4	2	2	3	5	5	5	4	4	1	3	40	3.33
2. Football (Touch)	1	2	1	1	2	4	3	3	3	3	1	1	25	2.08
3. Hockey (Field)	1	3	1	1	2	4	4	3	3	2	1	3	28	2.33
4. Lacrosse	2	3	2	1	3	3	4	3	3	2	1	3	30	2.50
5. Rugby	2	4	1	2	3	5	3	3	2	2	1	3	31	2.58
6. Soccer	2	4	2	2	3	5	3	4	2	2	1	3	33	2.77
7. Softball	0	0	1	0	1	2	3	2	2	1	1	0	13	1.08
8. Speedball	2	3	1	1	3	4	4	3	2	2	1	3	29	2.42
9. Volleyball	1	2	2	1	2	4	4	3	2	4	2	3	29	2.42
10. Waterpolo	3	4	4	2	6	3	4	2	2	3	1	3	37	3.08

235

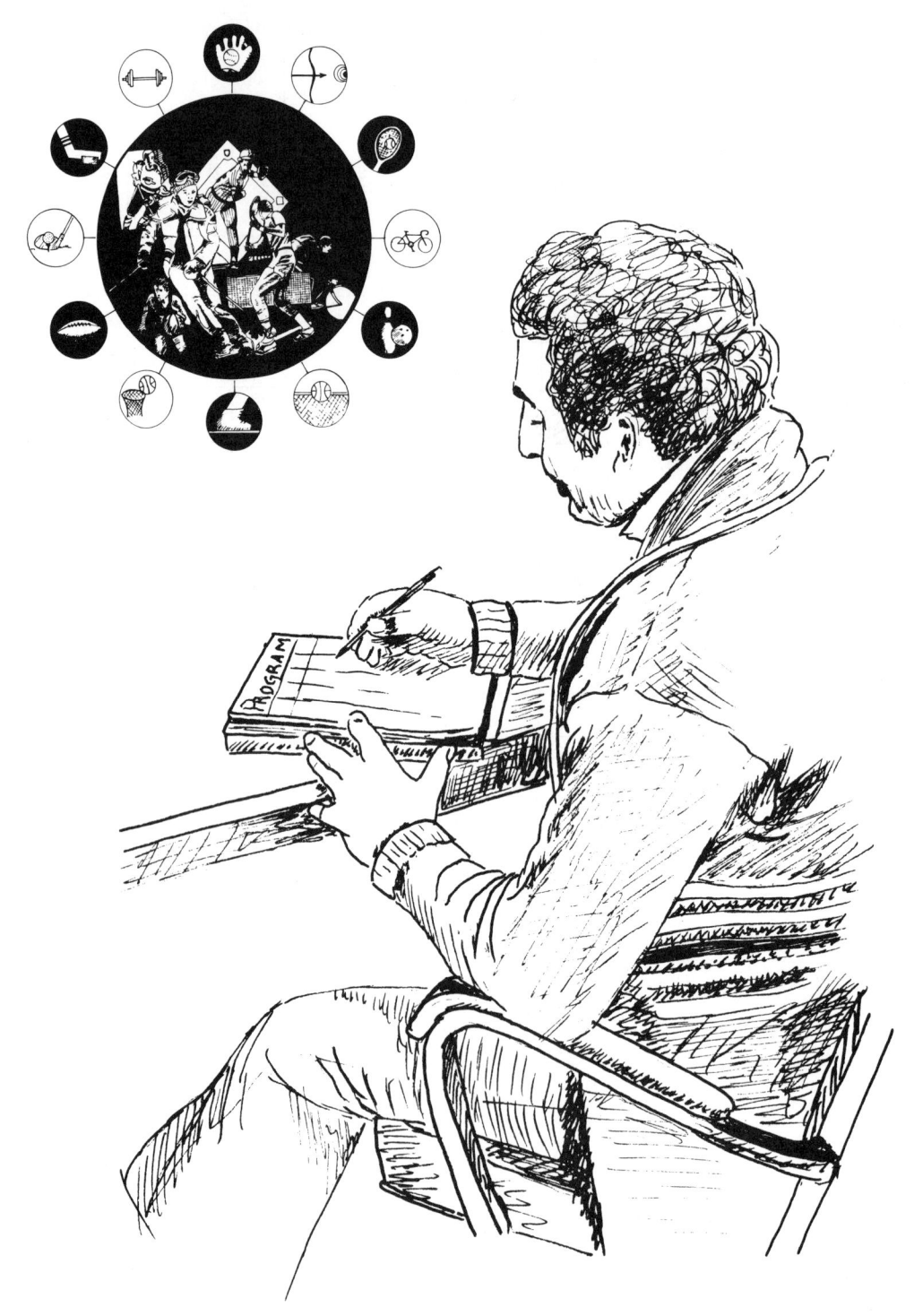

INDIVIDUALIZED ACTIVITY PROGRAM

PERSONAL APPRAISAL NO. 15
Individualized Activity Program

The development of your individualized lifetime activity program should be based upon understanding of self, knowledge of the conditioning process, and the goals which you seek to achieve.

Use your imagination and construct a sequence of activities which reflect your needs and interests. Incorporate variety to insure stimulation and enjoyment. As the program is made final, the primary emphasis should be on the acquisition and maintenance of those qualities which make life more meaningful.

Consider the analysis and implications of your previous "personal appraisals." On the basis of this information first select activities which reflect the concept of the "Golden Triangle." In addition include activities from the broad spectrum of sports. Make your choice after carefully analyzing the values of each sport in terms of your needs and interests.

With this recipe, mix the ingredients well. May the result serve you as a "Way of Life—For the Rest of Your LIfe."

Equipment and Facilities

    A. Results of Each Personal Appraisal 1–13.

    B. Creativity—Logic—Concentration.

Procedures

    A. Review and digest the results off all personal appraisals—know yourself!

    B. Select your activities and record them on Chart 1. Provide approximate percentage of time devoted to each activity in the total program. Determine and record your present skill level for each activity.
       (neophyte—beginner—intermediate—advanced—superior)

    C. Become more definitive by arranging activities into a sample weekly program on Chart 2. List the activities in sequence and show number of minutes devoted to each.

EVALUATION REPORT
Personal Appraisal No. 14

Name _____

Date _____

Lifetime Participation

I. *Title:* Individualized Activity Program

II. *Objectives:*

III. *Results:*

    A. Selection of Activities—

Chart I

	Areas of Concentration (make selection on the basis of the "personal appraisals")	Selection of Specific Activities	Minutes per Workout	Check Level of Intensity — High	Med.	Low	Frequency per Week
Golden Triangle	A. Flexibility						
	B. Aerobic/anaerobic						
	C. Progressive-resistance						
Spectrum of Sports	A. Individual						
	B. Small group						
	C. Large group						

B. Convert Chart I into a Weekly Schedule—

Chart II

Time of Day	Time Spent on Activity	Sunday	Monday	Tuesday	Wednesday	Thursday	Friday	Saturday

IV. *Analysis and Implications:*

    1. With your present responsibilities, circle the number of days per week you can include in your fitness program

       1 2 3 4 5 6 7

       State the average number of minutes that you will include in each exercise period.

       Minutes: _____

    2. What would be the minimum amount of time that you would insist be included in your weekly workout program regardless of other responsibilities:

       Days per week _____ Ave. min. per day _____

    3. State what you feel are the most important aspects of fitness in your personal program.

    4. Describe a minimal program of activity that you can recommend for your parents. (Base this program on their needs, interest and capabilities.)

    5. Describe legitimate circumstances or situations that might limit, reduce or detract from your ability to participate in an ideal program.

    6. In light of the above, describe adaptations that you could make in your program that would enable you to continue in an abbreviated manner, yet still keep fitness benefits.

THE END TO WHAT WE HOPE WILL BE "THE BEGINNING"

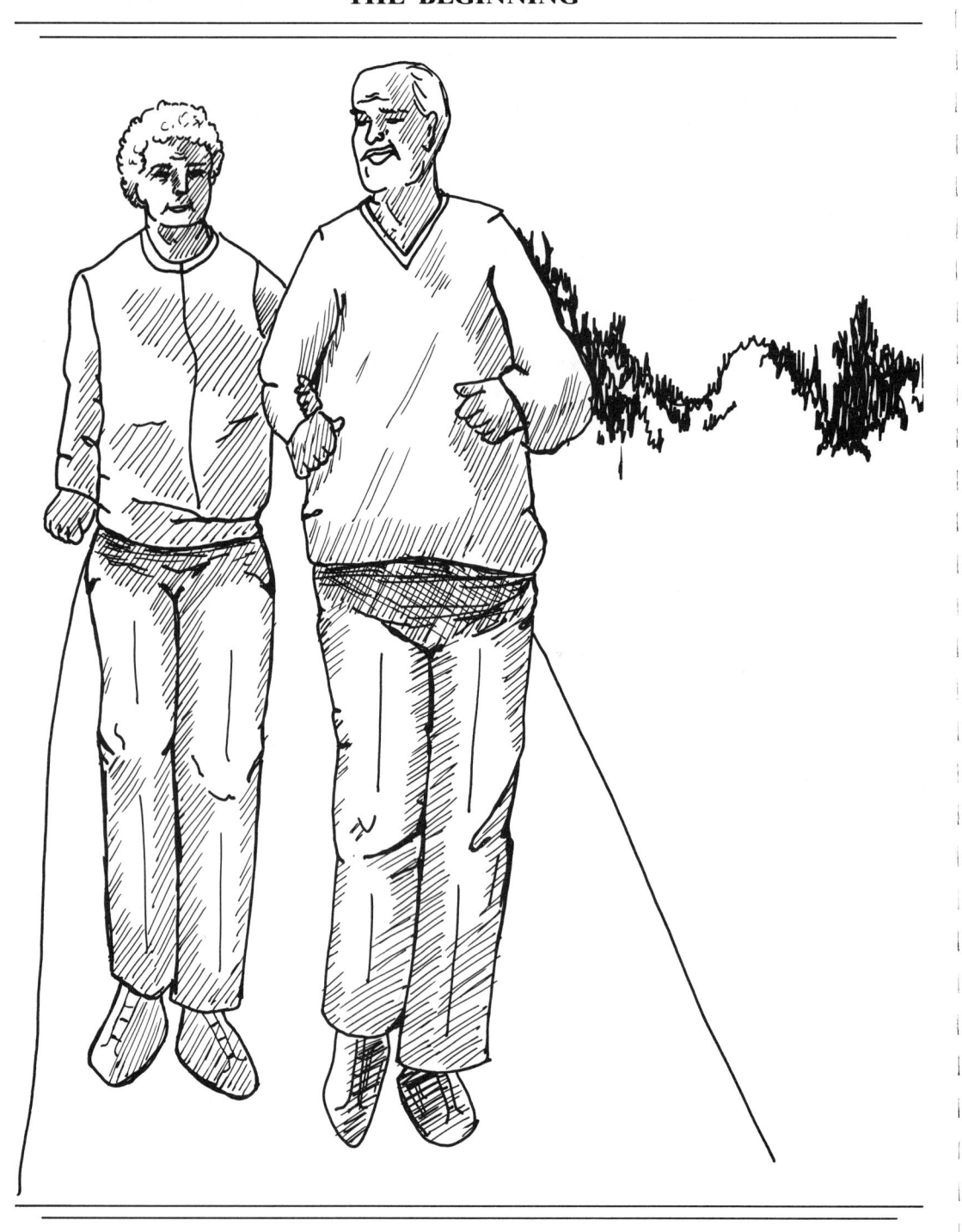

18
THE END TO WHAT WE HOPE WILL BE THE BEGINNING

There are so many reasons for becoming enthusiastic about pursuing the active life. We feel the important concepts have been stressed.

We are still, however, dealing with individuals who become motivated to participate for many different reasons:

As an example: We were trying to organize a Faculty/Staff Fitness Group on campus, and one afternoon at the lunchroom we encountered a Professor of Psychology. We began by discussing with him the possibility of his joining the fitness group. He was emphatic! He would have no part of it. We told him that rather than being so negative he should give us a chance to at least ennumerate the six important reasons as to why he should join us, to make fitness a "Way of LIfe." Somewhat facetiously we began:

Reason 1—"Being physically fit would extend and enhance your sex life!"

The Psychology Professor responded immediately by saying—"Never mind what reasons 2, 3, 4, 5, or 6 may be. Where do I sign??"

Ultimate Question

There are countless reasons for being physically active—you know how you feel! Everyone knows how you look! Regular exercise can improve your sense of well-being and your appearance! What do you intend to do about it, today, tomorrow, and in the future?

The Apprentice Period

Be prepared to expend time and effort in the acquisition of skill. During the learning phase you may become discouraged and react negatively. You may not want to appear inept in the activity and look foolish in the eyes of others, or you may feel the time necessary to develop skill is not worth the effort. You must resist this psychological barrier, for the apprentice period must be served if new skills are to be learned.

Once the apprentice period is accepted, developing proficiency in new sport activities becomes more enjoyable, since:

1. The conditioning process continues regardless of skill level.
2. The challenge of learning new skills can be truly enjoyable.
3. Identical elements can be transferred from one sport to another which enhances the learning process and reduces the apprentice period.
4. There is a wealth of wholesome competition at each respective skill level, from the novice to the expert.
5. As we become more highly skilled in a wide variety of sport activities, it becomes less difficult to remain physically active and enjoy a better state of life.

The apprentice period is the time necessary to:

1. Improve fundamentals.
2. Develop a high level of conditioning.
3. Test your skills in a variety of competitive situations.
4. Gain confidence through experience. Reduce the tendency to "choke." Example: There is a difference between perceived pressure while playing golf with a friend or with Jack Nicklaus as your opponent.
5. Maintain consistent performance.

The Myth of Chronological Age:

Many of the degenerative physical changes that can be attributed to aging are simply the result of inactivity. Unfit people age more quickly becuse they suffer from a deficiency of sufficient exercise with all its resultant benefits. There is strong evidence which demonstrates a correlation between inactivity and early aging. It is pointed out that some of the physical changes resulting from aging include decreased cardiac output and breathing ability, lower physical work capacity, loss of muscular strength and endurance, reduction in muscle tone and the accumulation of adipose tissue. The well-conditioned individual will experience these same changes which are usually attributed to aging if inactivity prevails for a relatively short period of time. Trained athletes become fat and flabby, not because they grow older, but because they stop exercising. This transformation is by no means due to aging, it is due to the fact that exercise has been discontinued, muscle tone has been lost and fat has been gained.

Beware of the Chronological Age Syndrome!

There can be no doubt that physical, motor, physiological, and psychological changes go on throughout the life span of men and women. During the growth period, these changes reflect greater development and effectiveness until maturity is reached. For a few years, these gains may be maintained. Then a gradual deterioration takes place through the middle years and into old age as the activities of the body and its physiological processes are slowed. It is difficult, however, to distinguish between the actual process of aging and such environmental influences as the amount of exercise, dietary and other health practices, tensions, human associations, mental attitude, and the like. The aging process is slowed when the individual exercises as a way of life; and the process is speeded when the individual is sedentary. To prove this point, regardless of an individuals age, enforced inactivity such as extended bed rest will induce many of the physiological deteriorations found in aging. It is well known that our astronauts experienced physical deterioration resulting from weightlessness and inactivity during space flights. In later flights instruments for exercising were installed in spacecraft and exercise regimens were prescribed for the occupants. All physiological processes of the body are affected by exercise.

While the nature, extent, and significance of physical and motor differences have been demonstrated for younger ages, they also can be demonstrated throughout the life span. Observe any group of elderly persons: some are tall, some are short; some are skinny, some are fat; some are strong, some are weak; some erect and some stooped; some are endomorphs, some are mesomorphs, some are ectomorphs; some are mentally alert, some are senile; some are aggressive, some are vacillating; some are extroverts, some are introverts; and on and on. Yet, despite the obvious, society clings to "chronological age" as the single most important criterion when decisions are made. The most obvious at the present time is the decision in reference to the age of retirement.

Just what does elderly mean? This country has had great elder statesmen in all walks of life: jurists, philosophers, athletes, educators, scientists, physicians authors, poets, historians, artists, musicians, humanists, industrialists, inventors, and many more. Let us recognize that each individual has inherent and acquired capabilities and that age alone should never be a deterrent to worthwhile accomplishments.

Everyone Can Be a Winner

We want everyone to become a winner! In a pure sense you will when you make the most of your life—living up to your true potential.

Embrace the concept of "preventive maintenance"

Condition the body so it is prepared for the rigors of daily living!

Condition the body to assist in warding off disease or to have the strength and vitality to better cope if illness should occur!

Condition the body to be better able to resist injury and to have greater recuperative powers if injury should occur!

Condition the body to delay the effects of aging!

Condition the body to better enjoy the "good" life!

Do not be easily discouraged in your quest for satisfaction and happiness throughout life. Some people who lack drive and motivation sit down and withdraw from life's opportunities. Not attempting to succeed is worse than failing. How boring it is to live in the gray twilight that knows neither brightness nor shadow, neither victory nor defeat.

Let your preparations for making the most of your life reflect your hopes and the wonder of your enterprise. Of this be sure, there is no free pass that will admit you to a full and satisfying life. If your effort appears to be tedious or irksome, recall your purpose and your vexations during your quest will seem trivial.

Embrace active living and experience all those wonderful changes that occur as a result of the conditioning process. Maintain and persist in your program as continual involvement will result in a personal metamorphosis with physical activity as a "Way of Life."

Ancient proverb: *"I have two doctors: my left leg and my right"*

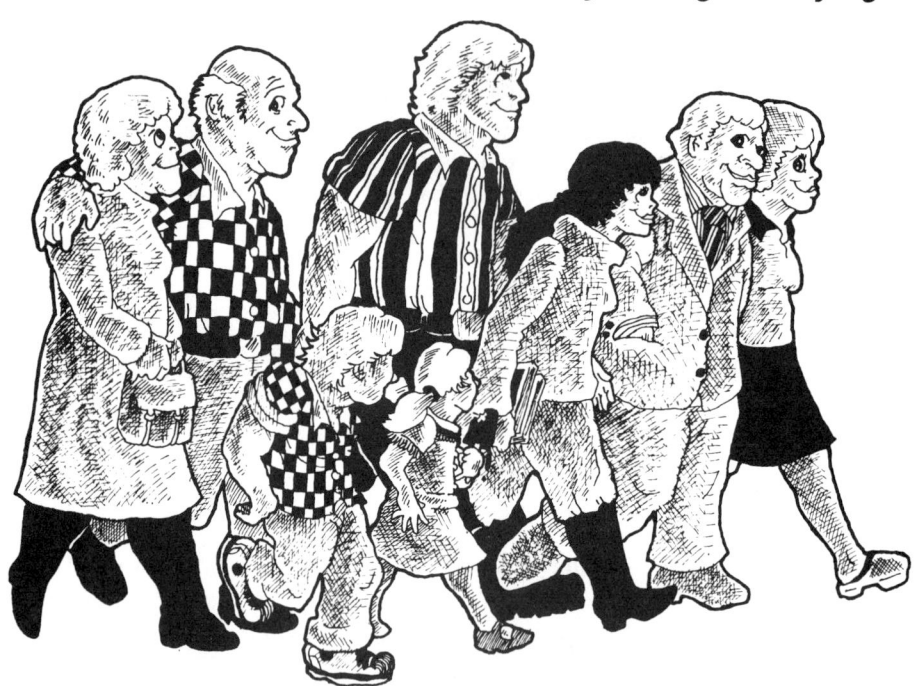

Start to experience the many benefits of *"active living"*
Begin by walking

BLOCK THE DEVIL

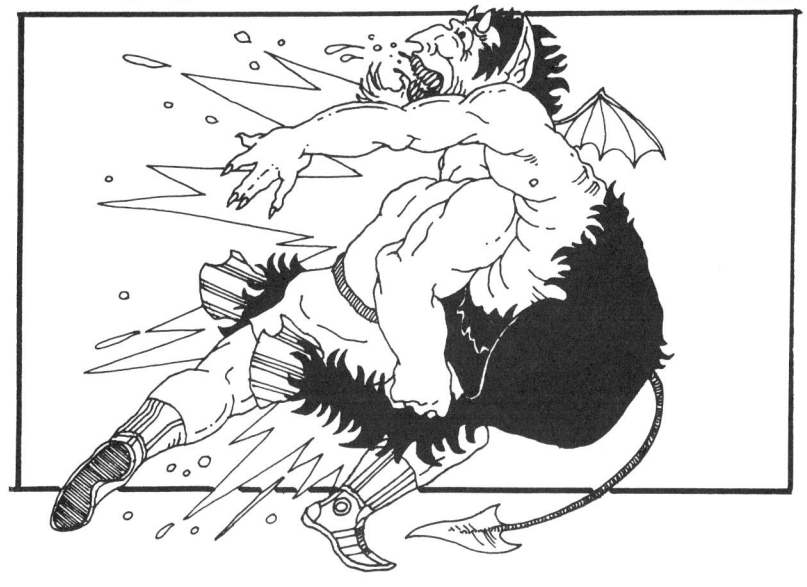

No. 18

No. 19

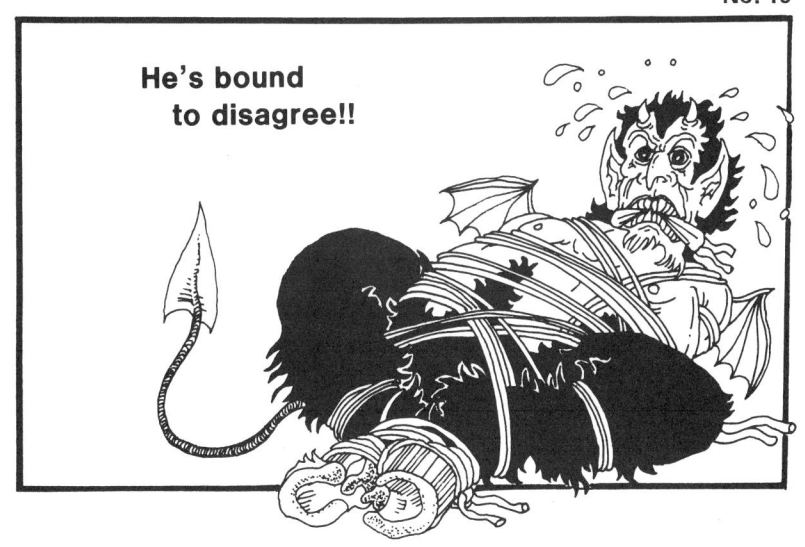

He's bound to disagree!!

GLOSSARY

Abdomen—The part of the body located between the thorax and pelvis.
Achilles—The calcaneal tendon, which is attached to the calcaneus.
Adipose Tissue—Fat or fat tissue.
Adrenalin—A hormone secreted by the adrenal gland. Produces the fight or flight syndrome.
Aerobic—In the presence of oxygen.
Aerobic Capacity—The ability to supply and utilize oxygen.
Agonist—The "prime mover" or the muscle that is directly engaged in the contraction that produces a desired movement.
Agility—The inherent ability to change direction quickly and efficiently.
Albumin—Simple heat-coagulable water-soluble proteins found in blood plasma or muscle.
Alimentary Tract—The alimentary canal, which is composed of the mouth, pharnyx, esophagus, stomach and the small and large intestines.
Alveoli—Very small terminal air sacs in the lungs in which gaseous exchange with the blood in the pulmonary capillaries occurs.
Amino Acid—The organic compounds from which protein is constructed.
Amphetamines— A stimulant to the central nervous system used in reducing fatigue and increasing the capacity for work.
Anaerobic—In the absence of oxygen.
Anabolic Steroid—A protein building hormone that has masculinizing properties.
Androgenic—Any substance that may produce masculinizing properties.
Antagonist—A muscle that exerts an action opposite to that of the prime mover or against muscle.
Antibodies—Substances produced by the body that destroys a specific pathogen (foreign material) after it has entered the body.
Artery—A vessel that carries blood away from the heart.
Arteriole—A very small branch of an artery.
Arteriosclerosis—Degenerative disorder of the blood vessels which affect arterial walls and cause high blood pressure and heart attacks.
Arthritis—Inflamation of the joints due to an infectious, metabolic or constitutional cause.
Articulation—Any joint or meeting place of bones.
Atherosclerosis—Hardening of the arteries resulting in high blood pressure. This is one form of arteriosclerosis.
Atrophy—The wasting away of tissue; a decrease in the size of a body part.
Balance—The maintenance of equilibrium.
Ballistic Stretching—Stretching movements occurring quickly and in short bursts.
Biceps—Biceps brachii; the muscle that flexes the forearm.
Bi-ped Position—Standing on two feet.
Blood Pressure— The driving force that moves the blood through the circulatory system. Pressure of the blood against the arterial walls.
Blood Volume—The amount of blood contained within the circulatory system.
Body Mechanics—The position of the body and its segments during movement and at rest.

Bronchiole—A small branch of bronchus (one of the two branches of the trachea).
Bursa—A fluid-containing sac lined with synovial membrane.
Calcification—The process by which calcium salts are deposited in the bone or cartilage.
Calorie—A unit of work that is equal to the amount of heat required to raise the temperature of one gram of water one degree centigrade.
Capillary—A network of small vessels located between the arteries and veins in which exchanges of vital substances occur between tissue and blood.
Capillary Bed—A system of interrelated parts which consist of the arterioles, venules and smaller vessels between them.
Carbohydrate—Any of a group of chemical compounds, which include sugars, starches and cellulose, which contain carbon, hydrogen and oxygen only. One of the basic and essential nutrients.
Carbon Dioxide—Gaseous waste product of metabolism.
Cardiac Output—The amount of blood pumped by the heart in one minute.
Cardio-respiratory—The system that incorporates both the respiratory and circulatory systems.
Cardio-respiratory Capacity—The ability of the heart vascular system and lungs to respond to life's requirements for energy, nutrition and waste removal.
Cardio-respiratory Endurance—The ability of the lungs and heart to take in and transport sufficient amounts of oxygen to the working muscles, allowing activities that involve large muscles to be performed over long periods of time.
Cardio-respiratory Fitness—Having a sound and healthy cardio-respiratory system.
Cardiovascular—Incorporating the heart and blood vessels.
Carotid Artery—A major artery located on each side of the neck allowing blood to flow from the aorta to the head.
Cell—The basic structural and functional unit of all organisms.
Cerebellum—That part of the brain that is concerned with the coordination of movements.
Chemicals—In anatomy, all substances that enter the circulatory system.
Chronological Age—Age of individuals based purely on the total number of years of life.
Circulatory System—Primarily consisting of the blood, heart and vascular bed.
Concentric—Muscular contraction in which fibers shorten during work.
Coordination—Efficient movement during the completion of a motor task.
Core Program—The central or basic program.
Coronary—Relating to the coronary arteries or veins of the heart. Also referring to heart attack.
Creatine Phosphate—A nitrogenous substance found in muscles.
Diaphragm—The muscle division between the thorax and the abdomen.
Diastolic Blood Pressure—The blood pressure during the relaxation phase of the heart cycle.
Diuretic—Tending to increase the flow of urine from the body.
Dynamic Balance—Maintaining equilibrium during movement.
Dynamic Lung Volume—The amount of air in the lungs during movement.
Dynamometer—An instrument which measures mechanical force.
Eccentric—Muscular contraction in which fibers lengthen during work.
Ectomorph—A body type characterized by linearity, fragility and delicacy of the body.
Endomorph—A body type characterized by roundness and softness of the body.
Enzyme—A protein substance that speeds up chemical reactions.
Ergogenic Aid—Any factor that improves the performance of work.
Extension—A motion that increases the angle between two joints.

External Respiration—The passing of the oxygen from the alveoli of the lungs into the capillaries and carbon dioxide passing from the capillaries of the lungs into the alveoli.
Fat—A compound that contains glycerol and fatty acids. One of the basic foodstuffs.
Fibrinogen—A soluble blood protein which is converted to insoluble fibrin during clotting.
Flexibility—Range of motion of a joint.
Flexion—A motion that increases that angle between two bones.
Force—The amount of strength or tension exerted.
Gas Transport—The physiological function of movement of molecules of gas throughout the body.
Gastrocnemius—The largest muscle of the calf, helps flex and extend the foot.
Girth—The circumference of body parts or segments.
Globulin—Any of a class of simple proteins, such as Myosin.
Glucose—Sugar.
Gluteal Region—The area comprising the buttocks.
Glycogen—An insoluable starch like substance.
Groin—Juncture of the lower portion of the abdomen and the inner portion of the thigh.
Hamstring—The muscle group that flexes the knee and extends the thigh.
Hemoglobin—A conjugated protein respiratory pigment located in the red blood cells.
Horizontal Plane—A flat and level surface that is parallel to the ground.
Hormone—A chemical substance that is secreted by an endocrine gland, which is absorbed into the blood and influences growth, development and function in some part of the body.
Hyperextension—Extension beyond the natural anatomic position.
Hypertrophy—The enlargement of a muscle.
Iliac Crest—The upper portion of the hipbone.
Intercostal Muscles—Those muscles that control inspiration and expiration.
Internal Respiration—When oxygen and carbon dioxide are exchanged between the cells and the capillaries.
Isokenetic—Maximum resistance over a complete range of motion.
Isometric—During muscle contraction joint angles remain unchanged and no movement of a body part results.
Isotonic—During muscle contraction angles of joints change and movement of body parts result.
Kilocalorie—The quantity of heat that is necessary to raise the temperature of one kilogram of water, one degree centigrade.
Kyphosis—Exaggerated curvature of the thoracic vertebra which sometimes results in a hunchback appearance.
Lactic Acid—A metabolite of the lactic acid system, which results in fatigue, and is due to the incomplete breakdown of glucose.
Latissimus Dorsi—The broad muscles of the back that function in adducting, extending and rotating the humerus in a medial direction.
Ligament—A band of white fibrous tissue that connect bones.
Lipids—Fats and fatlike substances.
Locomotive—The ability to move independently from one place to another.
Lordosis—An abnormal anterior convexity of the spine; known as swayback.
Mesomorph—A body type characterized by a square body with hard, rugged and prominent musculature.
Metabolic Rate—The rate of metabolism, the chemical and physical process continually going on in the living organism.

Metabolism—The process by which assimilated food is built up into protoplasm and protoplasm is used or broken down.

Metamorphosis—The change of physical form, substance or structure.

Motor Unit—An individual motor nerve and the muscle fibers it innervates.

Movement Efficiency—Motion utilizing the least amount of energy.

Movement Time—The amount of time in which a body or its extremities can move from one position to another.

Muscle Boundness—A imbalanced development of strength between the antagonist and agonist muscle in which a loss of flexibility occurs.

Muscular Endurance—The ability of the muscle tissue to persist in performing submaximal contractions.

Muscle Fiber—Threadlike structures of muscle that have contractive properties.

Muscle Tone—The normal tension or responsiveness of a muscle to stimuli.

Muscular Contraction—The shortening of muscle which produces force or tension.

Muscular Strength—The ability of muscle to create force or tension.

Muscular System—The skeletal muscular system which is composed of skeletal muscular tissue and connective tissues that make up the individual muscles.

Non-locomotive—The body located in a stationary position without moving from one place to another.

Neophyte—A novice or beginner.

Nervous System—The bodily system that interprets and receives stimuli and transmits impulses to the effector organs.

Neuron—A motor nerve.

Obesity—Having an excessive amount of stored fatty tissue.

Overload Principle—Exposing the muscular, articulation and cardio-respiratory systems to additional or increased work and stress than is normally experienced.

Oxygenation—To supply with oxygen.

Oxygen Deficit—The time period during exercise in which the level of oxygen consumed is below that necessary to supply the amount of ATP required for exercise.

Oxygen Uptake—Oxygen absorption into an organism.

Peripheral Blood Distribution—Blood circulation at or near the surface of the body.

Plateau Tendency—Cessation of progress in an exercise or program.

Platelet—Minute protoplasmic discs of vertebrate blood that assist in the clotting of blood.

Plumb Line—A weighted line used to determine verticality.

Posture—The bearing or position of the body.

Power—The ability to exert maximum muscular force through distance in the shortest amount of time.

Progressive Resistance—Overloading the muscle while exposing it to increased workloads.

Progressive Resistance Exercise—A logical sequence in the amount of resistance encountered by a muscle or muscle group throughout the range of motion.

Prone Position—Lying in the face down position.

Protein—A substance containing amino acids. One of the basic nutrients.

Psychosomatic—Pertaining to the influence of the mind on the body.

Ptosis—A dropping or downward displacement of an organ or body structure.

Quadraceps—A muscle group that functions in extending the knees and flexing the thighs.

Reaction Time—The amount of time necessary to initiate a response to a stimulus.
Recovery Time—The amount of time necessary for the body to regain normal condition after exercise.
Red Blood Cell—The cell that carries oxygen to the tissue.
Repetition—The number of times a motion is repeated during a specific exercise.
Resting Heart Rate—The heart rate while the body is at rest.
Sacro-lumbar Joint—The joint between the sacrum and the lumbar portion of the spinal column.
Scapula—The shoulder blade.
Scoliosis—An abnormal sideways curvature from the normal vertical line of the spine.
Set—The number of times a particular exercise is performed during a training session.
Serum Cholesterol—A number of a group of compounds known as sterols that are produced by the body and are found in the circulatory system.
Skeletal Muscle—A part of the total muscular system.
Skeletal System—The framework of bones that provides protection for our organs and allows movement.
Skinfold Calipers—A device used to measure body fat.
Specificity of Training—The principle of training in which specific training effects result from a specific type, method or style of exercise.
Speed—The amount of time in which the body or its extremities can move from one position to another.
Stamina—Staying power or endurance.
Static Lung Volume—The amount of air in the lungs without movement of the body.
Static Stretching—Stretching movements that occur slowly and are held for periods of time.
Stationary Balance—Equilibrium when in a fixed position.
Steady State—The time period during which a physiological function remains at a constant value or state.
Stress Tolerance—The ability to withstand stress.
Stroke Volume—The amount of blood the left ventricle of the heart pumps per beat.
Subcutaneous—Pertaining to below the skin.
Submaximal—A level below the maximum.
Sugar Feeding—Also referred to as carbohydrate loading. Taking in large quantities of carbohydrates prior to endurance events for energy purposes.
Supine Position—Lying on ones back with the face pointing upward.
Systolic Blood Presssre—The blood pressure during the contraction phase of the heart.
Tendons—A core or band of fibrous connective tissue that attaches muscle to bone.
Threshold of Training—The minimum level of heart rate that will produce the training effect.
Thyroid—The endocrine organ that is located just below the larynx.
Triceps—The triceps brachii muscle that extends the forearm.
Trigleceride—An ester of glycerol that contains three ester groups.
Trunk—The human body exclusive of the appendages and head.
Uric Acid—The chief nitrogenous waste of all vertebrates.
Vascular Bed—The circulatory bed that is composed of the arteries, small arteries, arterioles and capillaries which lead to the tissues where the exchange of oxygen, carbon dioxide, nutrients and waste products occur.

Vascular System—The system of blood vessels throughout the body.
Vein—A vessel that carries blood to the heart.
Ventilation—The exchange of gases and circulation in the lungs that is basic to respiration.
Venule—A small vessel that conducts veneous blood from a capillary to a vein.
Vessel—A canal or tube in which body fluid is circulated.
Vertical Plane—A flat or level surface that is perpendicular to the ground.
Visceral System—The system of the internal organs of the body.
White Blood Cell—A blood cell that contains no hemoglobin and functions in fighting disease.

NOTES

NOTES